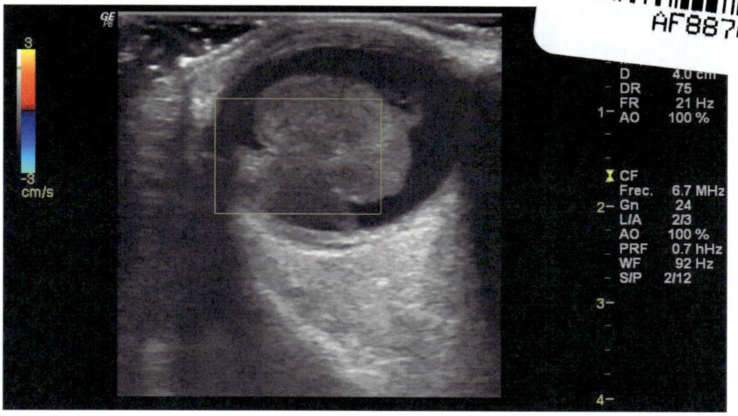

Echography in Ocular Pathology

Editors

Pedro Romero-Aroca

Ophthalmology Department
Hospital Universitario Sant Joan
University Hospital Sant Joan
Pere Virgili Health Research Institute [IISPV]
Rovira & Virgili University
Reus, Spain

&

Manuel Montero-Jaime

Ophthalmology Department
Hospital Universitario Sant Joan
University Hospital Sant Joan
Pere Virgili Health Research Institute [IISPV]
Rovira & Virgili University
Reus, Spain

CONTENTS

BIOGRAPHY

Pedro Romero-Aroca. Graduate in Medicine in 1983, form Universitat de Barcelona. Specialist in Ophthalmology since 1987, having studied in Hospital Valle Hebron de Barcelona. Doctor in Medicina from the Universitat Rovira i Virgili since 1995. Director of Ophthalmic Department of Ophthalmology of Hospital Universitario Sant Joan de Reus from 2000. Professor of Ophthalmology of Universitat Rovira i Virgili since 1997, responsible of as signature of Ophthalmology in the Docent Unit of Hospital Universitario Sant Joan de Reus from 2010, as a docent, he realized a total of 298 annually credits of formation at pregraduate and postgraduate students. Principal investigator of ophthalmic group in the Institut de Investigations Sanitaries Pere Virgili [IISPV]. His main areas of research are: diabetic retinopathy, telemedicine in ophthalmology and retinal images. Editorial board member of different journals including Diabetes Care. His publications include 76 indexed articles, one book about diabetic retinopathy screening by telemedicine, and 8 book chapters. The scientific activity includes a total of 97 communications in different national and international congresses. His assistential activity includes vitreous retinal surgeon of Hospital Universitario Sant Joan de Reus, expert in combined surgery cataract plus vitrectomy using as vitreous retinal equipments: Millennium since 2000, Stellaris PC since 2010.

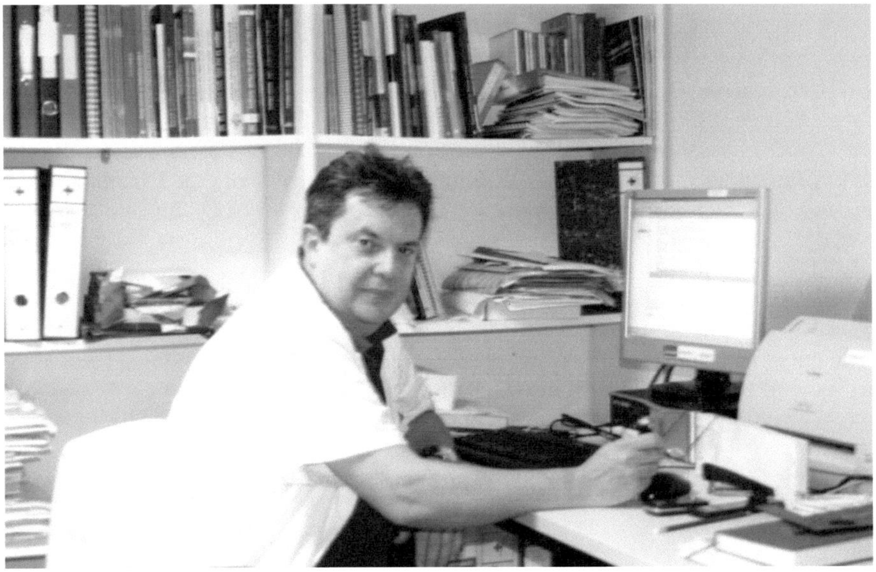

Manuel Montero-Jaime. Degree in Medicine by the University of Málaga in 1983. Specialist in Radiology since 1998, studying for his specialty in the Carlos Haya Hospital in Malaga. Doctor of Medicine from the Rovira i Virgili University in 2013. Senior radiologist at the University Hospital Sant Joan since 1999. Associate Professor of Radiology at the University Rovira i Virgili since 2013. His publications include six articles in refereed journals and one book chapter. The scientific activity includes a total of 60 papers in various national and international conferences. His care activity takes place in the University Hospital of Reus in the fields of Ophthalmology, Pediatrics and Musculoskeletal Radiology.

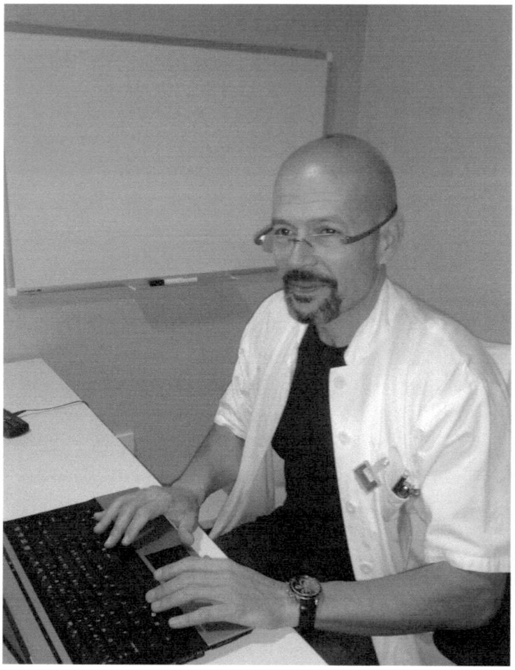

Francisco Ferrer-Jaime. Degree in Medicine by the University of Barcelona (1972). Doctor in Medicine and Surgery (Ph.D degree) by the University of Barcelona (1991). Master in Health Institutions (Autonomous University of Barcelona 2001-2002). Specialist in Radiology by University of Barcelona (1974). He has developed his clinical work in Hospital Valle Hebron (Barcelona) and the Hospital de la Esperanza (Barcelona). Director of Diagnostic Imaging Institute in the Hospital del Mar since 2002.

President of the Association of Radiologists of Catalonia from 1997 to 2013.

He has participated as principal author and coauthor communications in national and international conferences as well as publications in his specialty. Emphasizes its role in the implementation and quality control program for early detection of breast cancer in Barcelona.

About the eBook

The present book is the synthesis of the current concepts in ocular ultrasound examination. In chapters 1 and 2 the lector can learn the basis of the ultrasounds and know the different ultrasound systems as Color-Doppler echography, having a global knowledge about to management of ophthalmic pathology with ultrasounds. Chapter 3 describe the normal eye in ultrasound examination, lectors can acquire the knowledge of normal anatomy of the eye and its equivalents in ultrasounds. The anterior segment exploration by ultrasound is poorly known because the ultrasounds only permit us to observe anterior chamber and iris, but other techniques as BMU permit to examine the cornea, is in chapter 4 where we describe all these techniques. The most important indication for ultrasounds are the posterior segment examination, the lector can encounter in chapters 5 and 6 the more important pathologies which can be examined by ultrasounds. Ocular traumatisms are an important cause of blindness and the examination by ultrasounds is currently important, in chapter 7 the authors describe the different signs which we can encounter in traumatic ocular globe. Ultrasound and eye surgery is the topic of chapter 8, is very important to examine the eyes with ultrasounds previously to eye surgery in cases of poor fundus visualization, and in postoperative eye the ultrasounds have an important role. Finally the chapter 9 is dedicated to compere the ultrasounds with other image techniques, the computer tomography [CT] and magnetic resonance [MR] these two techniques are known in ophthalmology, but its importance is capital in some ocular pathologies, is in this chapter where lector can acquire a global vision of the eye examination with these the poorly known techniques.

FOREWORD

When the authors proposed the realization of this book thought it might be useful for both ophthalmologists, and radiologists, and while ophthalmologists hubs tend to perform their scans, mostly other practices of ultrasound an performed only by radiologists. We intend, therefore, that this work will be useful for clinical practice and understanding of the images obtained by ultrasound, being directed to these various health professionals and to all those to whom it may concern the interpretation of ocular ultrasound. The introduction of the application of ultrasound in ocular exploration started in 1956 with the first publication of Mundt and Hughues on the usefulness of echography in the diagnosis of intraocular tumors from that time, till now, there have been several improvements, especially, since the introduction of ultrasound contact type B introduced by Bronson in 1972 then, the need to calculate the power of intraocular lenses in cataract surgery, added a new impetus with the emergence of biometrics. The latest changes in the ultrasound scan of the eye with ultrasound techniques including use of different frequencies, can sometimes confuse and complicate their proper use, we will guide the reader and provide as much information as possible. It is the intent of the authors to make an extensive review of ultrasound applied to the eye examination, and making the reader to understand that ultrasound, is helpful, especially to compare the images obtained with those achieved with other diagnostic eye as computed tomography, magnetic resonance, 18FDG-PET/CT scans, and other ophthalmic techniques as retinography or the optical coherence tomography.

Francesc Ferrer Masip
President of Radiologists of Catalonia
Spain

PREFACE

The aim of the authors in this book is to explore the ultrasound of ocular globe. The echography of ocular images has been poorly known by ophthalmologist, due to the new imaging techniques such as optical coherence tomography [OCT], scanning laser and others, which have become the preference in the ocular exploration, relegating the ultrasound to cases with poor fundus visualization. The ocular echography is an excellent option to determine retinal lesions as in cases of ocular tumors. In this book, we resume the current knowledge about ocular ultrasound technique and its indications in ophthalmic pathology. Ocular echography is a basis in cases with media opacities, as when cataract or vitreous hemorrhage compare the correct vision of ocular fundus, mainly important in the preoperative cataract surgery, in order to diagnose possible retina pathologies that will affect the outcome of surgery. Furthermore the diagnosis of intraocular tumors as choroid melanoma is based on the echographic findings, as its differential diagnosis with other tumors as metastasis or hemangiomas, lectors encountered a chapter with all echographic findings for these pathologies. Currently, the introduction of Color-Doppler vascular examination, helps us in the diagnosis of ocular vasculopathies as arterial or venous occlusions, the authors dedicate a chapter to Color-Doppler ocular examinations. The most important objective of the authors is that the reader can have a global perspective of ultrasounds in ophthalmic examination, and can use this technique to ameliorate the ophthalmic patients management.

Pedro Romero-Aroca and Manuel Montero-Jaime
Ophthalmology Department
Hospital Universitario Sant Joan
University Hospital Sant Joan
Pere Virgili Health Research Institute [IISPV]
Rovira & Virgili University
Reus, Spain

List of Contributors

Ariadna Conejero-Olesti	Department of Ophthalmology, University Hospital Sant Joan, Rovira & Virgili University, Pere Virgili Health Research Institute, IISPV, Reus, Spain
Demetrio A Ramos-Dominguez	Department of Ophthalmology, Hospital Star Médica, Instituto de Seguridad y Servicios Sociales de los Trabajadores del Estado [ISSSTE], Mérida, Mexico
Francesc Ferrer Masip	Catalan Society of Radiology, Spain
Isabel Mendez-Marin	Department of Ophthalmology, University Hospital Sant Joan, Rovira & Virgili University, Pere Virgili Health Research Institute, IISPV, Reus, Spain
Javier Reyes-Torres	Department of Ophthalmology, University Hospital Sant Joan, Rovira & Virgili University, Pere Virgili Health Research Institute, IISPV, Reus, Spain
Jose A Buil-Calvo	Department of Ophthalmology, Hospital Santa creu i Sant Pau, Universidad Autonoma de Barcelona, Barcelona, Spain
Manuel Montero-Jaime	Department of Radiology, University Hospital Sant Joan, Rovira & Virgili University, Pere Virgili Health Research Institute IISPV, Reus, Spain
Marc Baget-Bernaldiz	Department of Ophthalmology University Hospital Sant Joan, Rovira & Virgili University, Pere Virgili Health Research Institute, IISPV, Reus, Spain
Monica Llagostera-Serra	Department of Ophthalmology, University Hospital Sant Joan, Rovira & Virgili University, Pere Virgili Health Research Institute, IISPV, Reus, Spain
Nuria Soler	Department of Ophthalmology, University Hospital Sant Joan, Rovira & Virgili University, Pere Virgili Health Research Institute, IISPV, Reus, Spain
Pedro Romero-Aroca	Department of Ophthalmology, University Hospital Sant Joan, Rovira & Virgili University, Pere Virgili Health Research Institute, IISPV, Reus, Spain
Victor Perez-Riverola	Radiology Department, University Hospital Sant Joan, Rovira & Virgili University, Pere Virgili Health Research Institute, IISPV, Reus, Spain

CHAPTER 1

Ultrasonic Ocular Systems

Manuel Montero-Jaime[1,*], Ariadna Conejero-Olesti[1] and Pedro Romero-Aroca[2,*]

[1]Department of Radiology, [2]Department of Ophthalmology, University Hospital Sant Joan, Rovira & Virgili University, Pere Virgili Health Research Institute, IISPV, Reus, Spain

Abstract: The ultrasound in ophthalmology took an important place, with multi-frequency linear probe between 15 to 18 MHz, with higher definition than the old 7 MHz probe. This chapter describes the different types of ultrasound techniques, described the poorly used A-mode echography, and with reference to Color-Doppler ultrasound, and its normal ocular values.

Keywords: Ultrasound, ocular echography, Color-Doppler, ocular artifacts, A-Mode echography, B-Mode echography.

INTRODUCTION

Scanning is made with multi-frequency linear probe between 15 to 18 MHz (Fig. **1**). The patient is placed supine with head in neutral position, eyelids closed and the gaze centered (Figs. **2**, **3**). After applying gel to perform sagittal and axial planes, overpressure on the ocular globe must be avoided, particularly in situations of ocular trauma and for Doppler study performing. A key aspect of ultrasound is its dynamic capability, which allows assessing the displacement of intraocular structures and their relation to the different eye layers. This can be achieved by asking the patient to mobilize the ocular globe in different planes of space. Another relevant aspect is the increase in gain relation. This increase makes the pathological findings more remarkable, particularly the membranes and vitreous bands.

1. Ocular Ultrasound Directions

Ultrasound examination is a safe, inexpensive and quick method. Even in situations in which the CT and MRI are superior for diagnosis, mainly from the

***Corresponding author Manuel Montero-Jaime:** Hospital Universitario Sant Joan, Avda. Doctor Josep Laporte 1 Reus, Spain; E-mail: mmontero@grupsagessa.com
Pedro Romero Aroca: Hospital Universitario Sant Joan, Avda. Doctor Josep Laporte 1 Reus, Spain; E-mail: pormero@grupsagessa.com

Pedro Romero-Aroca and Manuel Montero-Jaime (Eds.)

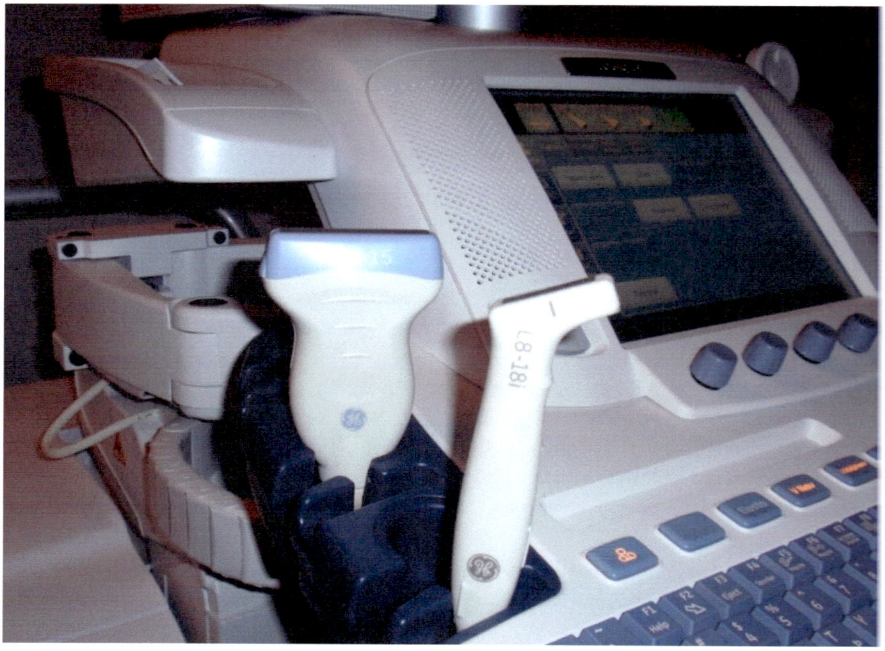

Figure 1: Probes of 15 [largest] and 12 [short] MHz.

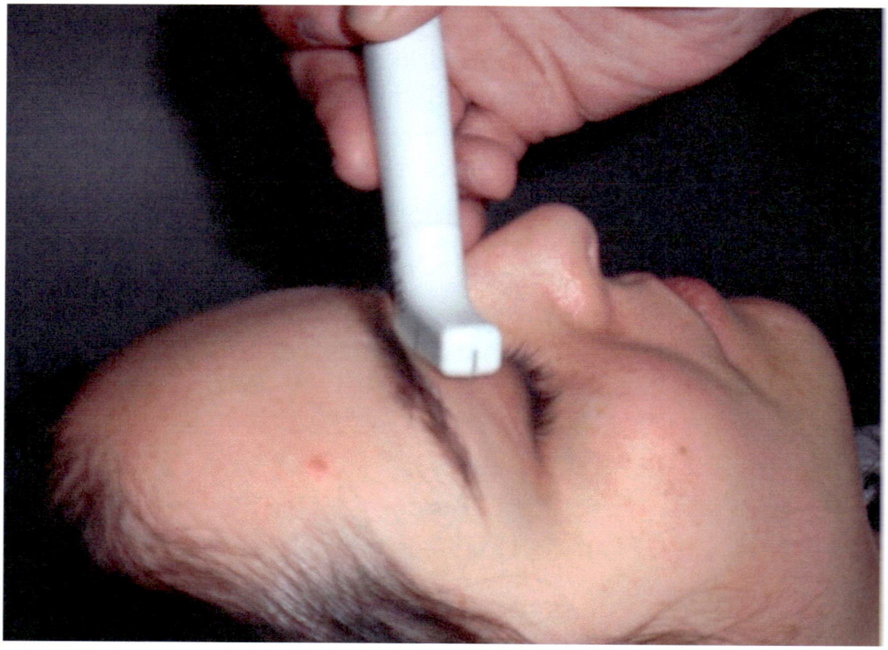

Figure 2: Exploration across closed eyelids with a 18 MHz probe. The patients should regard in front.

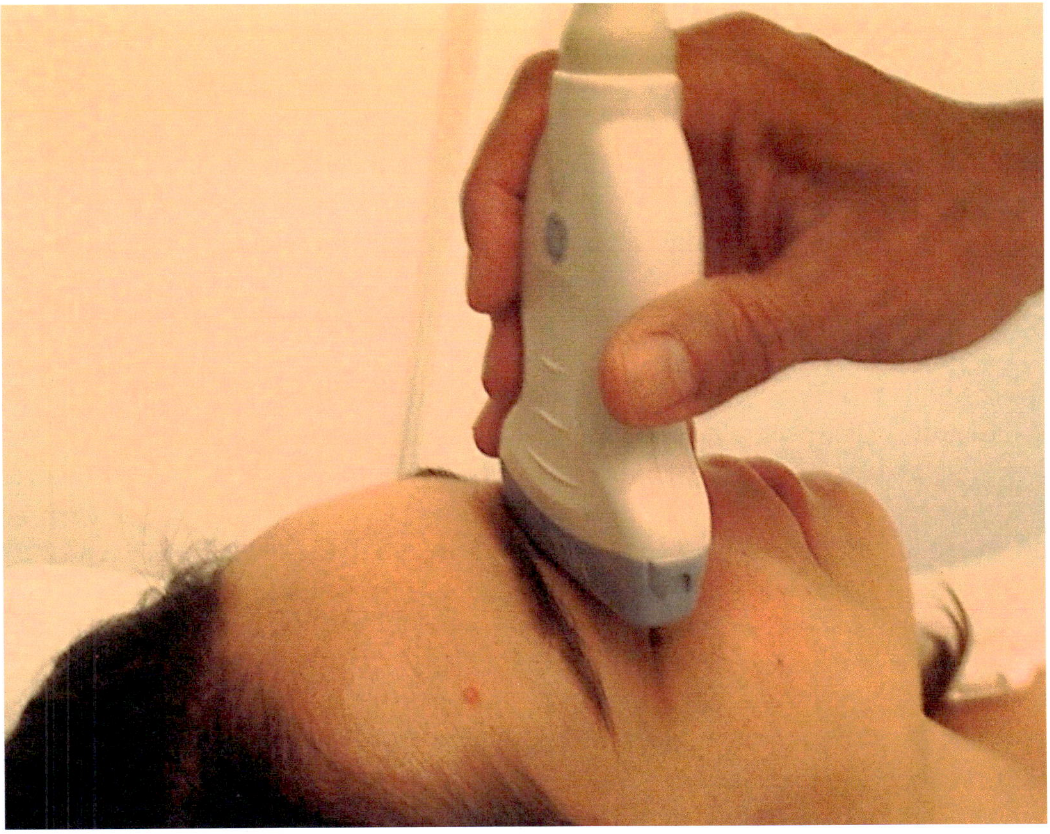

Figure 3: Technique of echography across closed eyelids, with a 15 MHz probe. The patients should regard in front.

orbital pathology, as we shall see in later chapters, ultrasound could be a suitable method for monitoring:

1) Media opacities
2) Vitreous opacities
3) Suspicion of intraocular tumor
4) Trauma
5) Intraocular foreign body
6) Monitoring of postoperative intraocular surgery

DOPPLER COLOR ULTRASOUND

The applications of Color-Doppler in the study of the eye are manifold, not only is a complementary technique to ultrasound B mode, but a first indication for exploration in intraocular and orbital vascular disorders [1]. In the literature there are several references to the usefulness of Color-Doppler mode B in cases of retinal detachment and differentiation of retinal membranes anchor; fibrovascular proliferations, especially in patients vitrectomized, and in general, the assessment of intraocular lesions, both for diagnoses and assessment of treatment response [2-4].

The scanning technique is similar to mode B for patient positioning and linear probe. The transducer frequency must be the lowest setting parameters, because of ocular slow flow and low resistance. Unlike the vessels of large and medium caliber where it is possible to perform a morphological study and achieve parameters such as intima-media thickening, define the presence of plaques and their characteristics [5, 6], the eye echographic functional parameters only get referred to spectral analysis [systodiastolic velocities, resistance index, *etc.*]. The systolic values in the orbital vessels have been determined in several studies [7-10], the normal values are described in Table **1**. The Ophthalmic artery and central retinal artery are clearly identified in relation to the optic disc head (Fig. **4**). The posterior ciliary arteries are located temporary and nasal in relation with the optic disc head. Alterations in the Doppler study are introduced in further chapters.

Table 1: Normal resistance index, systolic and diastolic velocity in major orbital vessels

Vessel	Velocity ± SD [cm/second]
Systolic velocity ophthalmic artery	32.7±12.8
Diastolic velocity ophthalmic artery	7.0 ±0.7
Resistance index ophthalmic artery	0.75 ± 0.25
Systolic velocity central retinal artery	7.9± 2.1
Diastolic velocity central retinal artery	2.3± 0.6
Resistance index central retinal artery	0.70± 0.06
Systolic velocity ciliary arteries	7.2± 1.5
Diastolic velocity ciliary arteries	2.5± 0.6
Resistance index ciliary arteries	0.65 ±0.07
Maximum velocity central retinal vein	3.6 ±.8
Minimum velocity central retinal vein	2.4 ±0.8

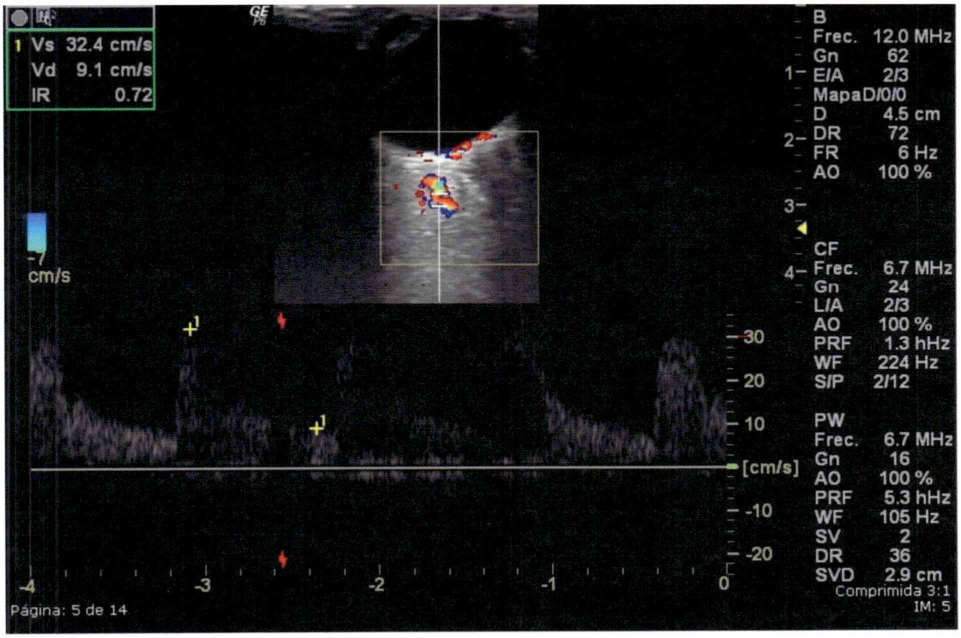

Figure 4: Typical color Doppler examination of ophthalmic artery, obtained values can be seen up and left. Down the echography we can observe the typical arterial pulse with systolic and diastolic peaks, signaled by yellow points.

TYPICAL ULTRASOUND ANATOMY

The assessment of the anterior pole of the ocular globe depends on the frequency of the transducer, thus the highest frequency the better spatial resolution. With the 15 MHz probe we can identify the cornea, the anterior chamber, the iris and ciliary body and posterior chamber and lens.

The normal cornea appears with two linear echogenic bands, parallel, separated by an anechoic interface. After the cornea has been identified, the anterior chamber appears with an anechoic aqueous humor, an image which also will be seen in the posterior chamber. The iris and ciliary body show a hypoechoic appearance with triangular morphology, whose apex is situated on both sides of the lens. The lens has an anechoic appearance with two echogenic bands of slight thickness, in relation to the anterior and posterior capsules. After the lens lies the anechoic vitreous chamber whose outer limits from internal to external are the retina, uvea and sclera, those which cannot differentiate trough a standard echography study. In the apex of the posterior pole of the eye, is easy to identify the optic nerve head, which has a markedly hypoechoic tubular structure (Fig. **5**).

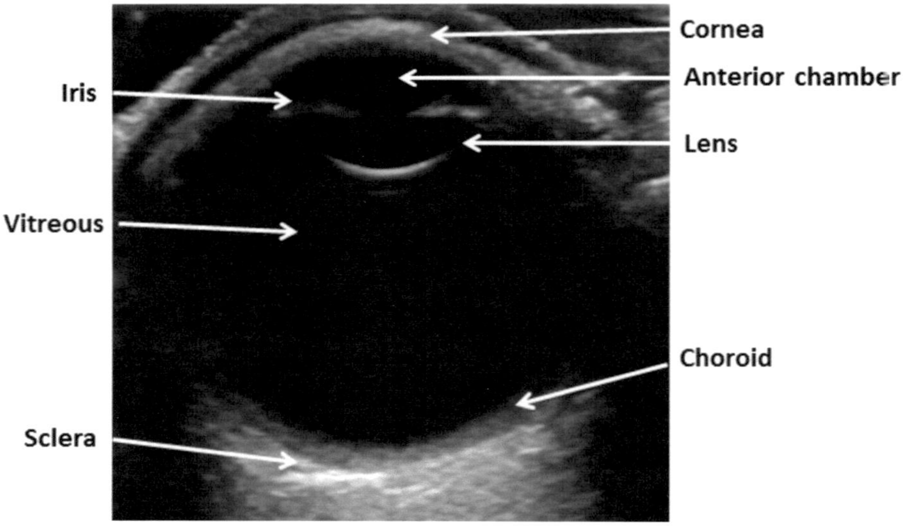

Figure 5: Description of ocular structures observed with B-mode probe echography.

OCULAR ARTIFACTS

Some artifacts are derived from the physical properties of the ultrasounds as reverberation and refraction. The first appears as a reflection of the structures of the anterior pole in the vitreous cavity [*i.e.* the posterior lens capsule into the vitreous], whereas the latter are related to the transducer position with respect to the ocular structures and disappear with changes in the position of it. In cases of therapeutic intraocular procedures such as injection of gas or silicone products generally used in surgery of retinal detachment, the artifacts are a significant limitation for fundus examination. If gas has previously injected, seated position could allow assess the patient's fundus, whereas the presence of oily materials prevents proper ultrasound examination of the ocular globe, in these cases MRI is particularly useful.

OTHER ULTRASOUND TECHNIQUES: A-MODE ECHOGRAPHY

Currently A-mode ultrasound has been poorly used. This technique was used extensively before B-mode ultrasound advances [11], when B-mode probes are of 7 MHz, although it was the basis for ocular biometry, currently has been poorly used.

The ultrasound image with A-mode probes is obtained applying the probe at the center of the cornea (Fig. **6**), perpendicular to anterior lens surface. The different echogenic surfaces [cornea, anterior lens surface, posterior lens surface and retina-sclera complex] produce peaks in the echogram [12]. Currently the A-mode echography have poorly used, and only in intraocular tumors permit us to suspect the presence of ocular melanomas [13]; and to measure the anterior-posterior axial length, a data essential to obtain the intraocular lens power after determination the corneal curvature with oftalmometer.

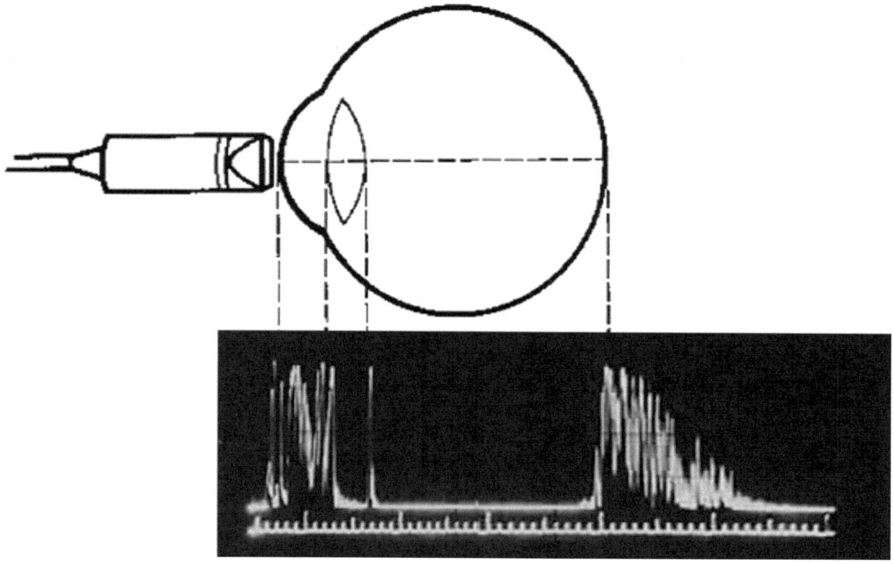

Figure 6: Echography with A-Mode probe, we observe the different echoes: Cornea, anterior lens surface, posterior lens surface and sclera echo, with the vitreous cavity with achogenic image.

CONCLUDING REMARKS

The 15 to 20 MHz echographies permit us to observe the globe structure, in a multiple of ocular pathologies. The A-mode echography has been reduced to melanoma diagnosis and for ocular biometry. Currently only B-mode echography are extended in the ocular examination.

ACKNOWLEDGEMENTS

Declared None.

CONFLICT OF INTEREST

The authors confirm that this chapter contents have no conflict of interest.

REFERENCES

[1] Lorente-Ramos RM, Armán JA, Muñoz-Hernández A, *et al.* US of the eye made easy: a comprehensive how-to review with ophthalmoscopic correlation. Radiographics. 2012; 32[5]: 175-200.

[2] Herwig MC, Löffler KU, Wells JR, *et al.* Clinico-pathological correlations: posterior compartment of the eye and orbit. Klin Monbl Augenheilkd. 2012; 229: 705-15.

[3] Harris A, Kagemann L, Cioffi G. Assessment of human ocular hemodynamics. Surv Ophthalmol 1998; 42: 509.

[4] Braband K, Kerty E, Jakobsen JA. Contrast enhanced ultrasound Doppler examination of the retrobulbar arteries. Acta Radiol 2001; 42: 135.

[5] Alonso-Villaverde C, Coll B, Parra S, *et al.* Atherosclerosis in patients infected with HIV is influenced by a mutant monocyte chemoattractant protein-1 allele. Circulation 2004; 110: 2204-9.

[6] Coll B, Parra S, Alonso-Villaverde C, *et al.* The role of immunity and inflammation in the progression of atherosclerosis in patients with HIV infection. Stroke 2007; 38: 2477-84.

[7] Kaiser HJ, Shötzau A, Stumpfig D, *et al.* Blood flow velocities of the extraocular vessels in patients with high-tension and normal-tension primary open-angle glaucoma. Am J Ophthalmol 1997; 123: 320.

[8] Lieb WE. Color-Doppler imaging of the eye and orbit. Radiol Clin North Am 1998; 36: 1059.

[9] Williamson TH, Baxter GM, Pyott A, *et al.* A comparison of Color-Doppler imaging of orbital vessels and other methods of blood flow assessment. Graefes Arch Clin Exp Ophthalmol 1995; 233: 80.

[10] Arai T, Numata K, Tanaka K, *et al.* Ocular arterial flow hemodynamics in patients with diabetes mellitus. J Ultrasound Med. 1998; 17: 675-81.

[11] Buschmann W. On ultrasonic measurement of the axial length of the eye. Klin Monbl Augenheilkd. 1964; 144: 801-15.

[12] Gernet H. Biometry of the eye by means of ultrasound. Klin Mol Augenheilk. 1963; 146: 863-74.

[13] Buschmann W, Goder G. Bilateral malignant melanoblastoma of the choroid. Albrecht Von Graefes Arch Ophthalmol. 1964; 167: 225-38.

CHAPTER 2

B-mode Ultrasound of the Normal Eye

Manuel Montero-Jaime[1,*], Pedro Romero-Aroca[2,*] and Victor Perez-Riverola[1]

[1]Department of Radiology, [2]Department of Ophthalmology, University Hospital Sant Joan, Rovira & Virgili University, Pere Virgili Health Research Institute, IISPV, Reus, Spain

Abstract: The ultrasound in ophthalmology held an important place, with multi-frequency linear probe being between 12 to 15 MHz, an obviously higher definition than the old 7 MHz probe. This chapter describes the different types of ultrasound techniques, with special reference to Color-Doppler ultrasound, and its normal ocular values.

Keywords: B-Mode echography, ocular globe anatomy, anterior segment echography, posterior segment echography.

INTRODUCTION

The orbit, basically a bone wall, gives protection to the ocular globe against injury. In addition, orbit cavity allows the extraocular muscles to undergo eye movements. The entire ocular globe is coated with a compartmentalized orbital fat and a fascia, and by the extraorbital muscles which are attached to each other through lateral extensions. The orbitary cone is fenestrated by several slots that communicate with the cranial cavity. The optic foramen at the orbital apex grants the ophthalmic artery and the optic nerve, access to the orbit. Nearby, there is the superior orbital fissure located in the external outer edge between the greater and lesser wings of the sphenoid bone. The Zinn ring is inserted in it that is the source of most extraocular muscles. Throughout this slot pass the three cranial nerves III, IV and VI; the first branch of the trigeminal nerve and in addition, the ophthalmic veins [1]. Finally, the sphenopalatine jaw recess communicates with the orbit pterygopalatine fossa which is situated in the external inferior edge of the orbit, whereby the trigeminal nerve maxillary branch passes together with the infraorbital artery. The anterior wall of the orbit is covered towards the eyelids

***Corresponding author Manuel Montero-Jaime:** Hospital Universitario Sant Joan, Avda. Doctor Josep Laporte 1 Reus, Spain; E-mail: mmontero@grupsagessa.com
Pedro Romero Aroca: Hospital Universitario Sant Joan, Avda. Doctor Josep Laporte 1 Reus, Spain; E-mail: pormero@grupsagessa.com

Pedro Romero-Aroca and Manuel Montero-Jaime (Eds.)

that provides protection above the ocular globe against the possible aggressions [light, wind, trauma, heat, *etc*]. The eyelids are two modified skin folds, being continuation of the integument of the face that seals the anterior base of the orbit when they are closed.

ORBITAL VASCULARIZATION AND ULTRASOUND APPLICATIONS

The ocular globe blood supply depends on the ophthalmic artery, which arises as the first branch of the internal carotid just as the vessel emerges from the cavernous sinus. Due to this particularity, the ophthalmic artery is the first vessel to be affected because of a blood debit, a condition that could be detected by an ultrasound carotid assessment. The ophthalmic artery enters the orbit through the optic foramen, below and on the outer orbit, and thence horizontally forward, beneath the lower border of the superior oblique muscle. This winding trajectory, bending over the optic nerve all over the course, could lead to cause difficulty in performing the Color-Doppler ultrasound (Fig. **1**). Along its course the ophthalmic artery branches may be divided into an orbital group, which supplies the orbit and the surroundings tissues and the ocular branches for the ocular globe structures and extraocular muscles. As the ophthalmic artery approaches closely the posterior pole of the ocular globe the central retinal artery appears, which pierces the optic nerve and runs forward in the center of it. This makes its detection possible by using Color-Doppler ultrasound focused on the entrance of the optic nerve to ocular globe. Therefore, the study of the posterior ciliary arteries becomes interesting for certain diseases such as Down's syndrome or pseudoexfoliation syndrome. The short ciliary arteries supply the choroid coat and ciliary processes, and the long ciliary arteries form an arterial circle around the iris. The orbitary veins drain to ophthalmic veins in both upper and lower areas, and leave the orbit through orbital fissure. Their ultrasound assessment is of limited usefulness [2, 3].

OCULAR GLOBE

The ocular globe consists of three layers: cornea-sclera, uvea and retina (Fig. **2**). The outermost is formed by the cornea anteriorly and the sclera, fibrous opaque structure behind, which is pierced by the optic nerve. The middle layer is the vascular layer of the ocular globe and is called uvea. It has three different portions: the anterior uvea and iris with the pupil at its center; the intermediate uvea consisting of the ciliary body with the ciliary processes that hold the lens; and the posterior uvea also called choroid, that consists mainly of a dense

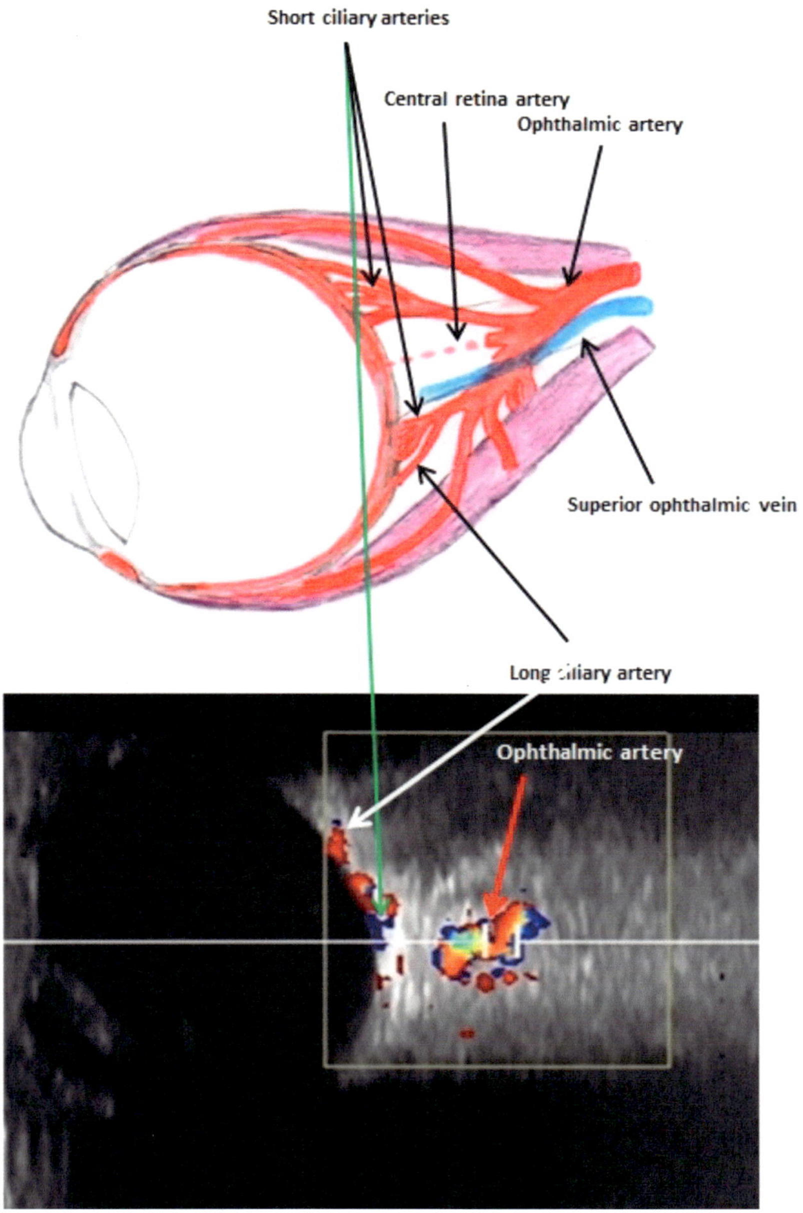

Figure 1: Up: schematic representation of orbital vessels, in a coronal orbital section. Down: ophthalmic artery observed in Color-Doppler in a same coronal orbital section.

capillary plexus which provides nutrients to the retina [4]. The inner layer is formed by the retina that covers the entire rear portion of the ocular globe and where the photoreceptors and the cells responsible for transmitting images to the brain are placed [bipolar cells and ganglion cells]. In the anterior third of the eye, the lens is suspended and fastened to the wall by the zonule eye, whose opacification is called a cataract, a condition that can be also studied using ultrasound. All these structures define a series of spaces occupied by two different kinds of fluids: the aqueous humor and the vitreous humor [1, 3].

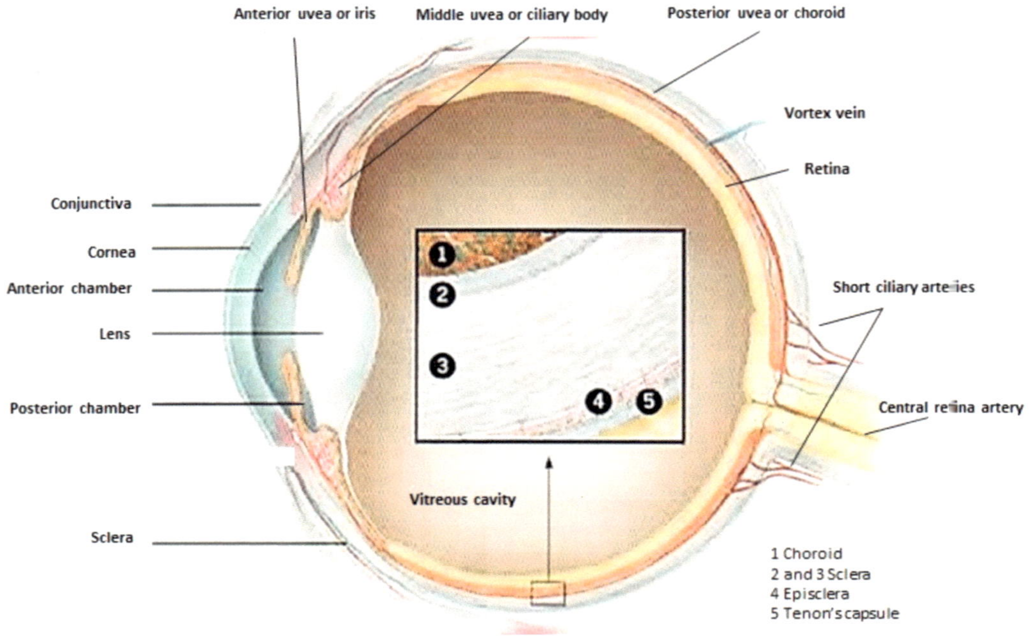

Figure 2: Anatomic ocular globe structures.

The aforementioned spaces are:

- The anterior chamber which is defined between the layer of the cornea [corneal endothelium] and the frontal surface of the iris and the crystalline lens at its center.
- The posterior chamber limits anteriorly by the posterior surface of the iris and the anterior lens surface behind. The aqueous humor completely fills the anterior and posterior chambers of the ocular globe.
- Vitreous cavity is limited by the back surface of the lens and its anterior zonules and the retina in the back side. The vitreous body fills this cavity.

These ocular structures allow to make an anatomical division of the ocular globe into two segments, the anterior segment that would be formed by the cornea, aqueous humor, iris and lens and the posterior segment consisting of the vitreous body, retina, choroid and sclera. Both segments have the level of translation by ultrasound scanning.

ANTERIOR SEGMENT ULTRASOUND FINDINGS

The anterior segment ultrasound focuses on those diseases that affect the anterior and posterior chambers, the iris and the crystalline lens and cornea [3]. The anterior chamber is very relevant in ultrasound. Typically, for an anechoic space, it is important to determine if there are areas that would be abnormally hyperechogenic. Also, ultrasound facilitates the assessment of the angle of the anterior chamber; which is formed by the posterior layer of the cornea and the anterior peripheral surface of the iris. Throughout this angle, the aqueous humor is removed and if it is closed at both sides [cornea and iris] it could lead to acute angle-closure glaucoma. The iris is an interesting structure to observe and is seen as a hyperechoic space that is in continuity with the wall of the ocular globe. In its center, we find the pupil, an anechoic space. The presence of increased thickness in the iris stroma, raises the possibility of a tumor at this level. The crystalline lens is formed by a series of concentric layers formed by collagen-like fibers which are called crystals and their parallel arrangement allows the passage of light through them. In ultrasonic assessment, crystalline lens appears as an anechoic space in the center of the pupil with a slightly hyper-echogenic line in the front and back. As the lens becomes cloudy, the anechoic image turns to hyper-echogenic (Figs. **3**, **4**). If subluxation or dislocation of the lens is present, lateral movement thereof is observed in the first case, or the lens is found within the vitreous cavity in the second case. The application of ultrasound also allows us to observe in cases of patients who underwent cataract surgery, the location and state of the intraocular lens (Fig. **5**). This prosthetic lens appears as a lenticular image [smaller in antero-posterior diameter than the crystalline lens] and is placed in the capsular bag [2].

POSTERIOR SEGMENT ULTRASOUND FINDINGS

The exploration of the posterior segment for helping the diagnosis of diseases of retina, choroid and sclera is actually the leading cause of ocular ultrasound requests. The vitreous cavity is occupied by the vitreous body which has an anechoic signal seen as a black area at the ultrasound assessment (Fig. **6**). The relevance of the vitreous lies in the examination of the possible opacities inside it

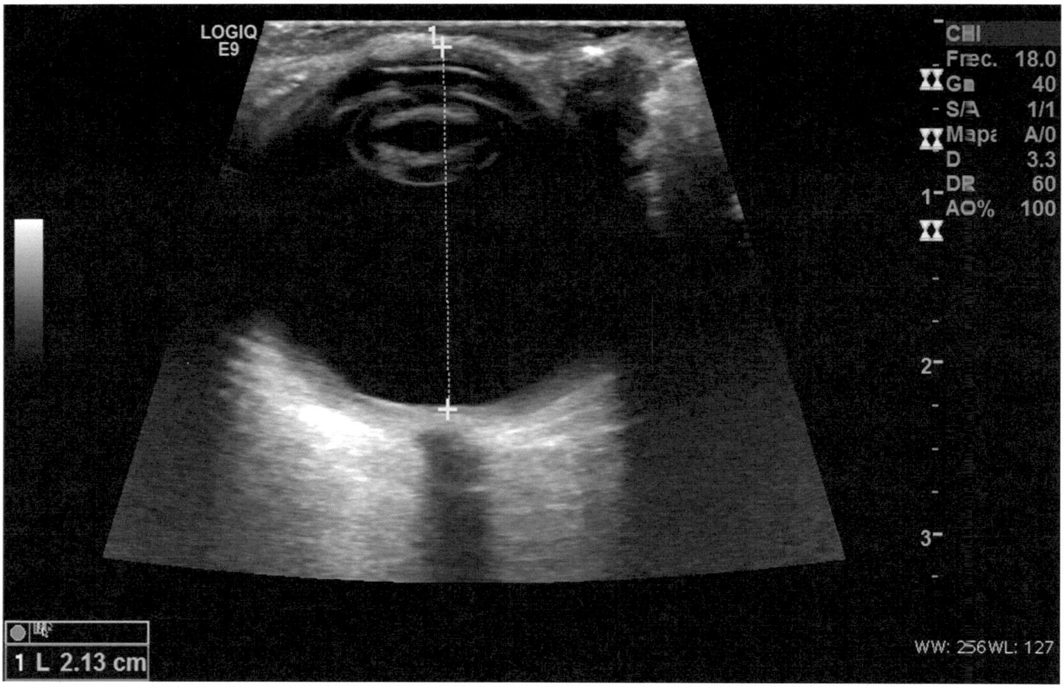

Figure 3: Cataract, axial length measure.

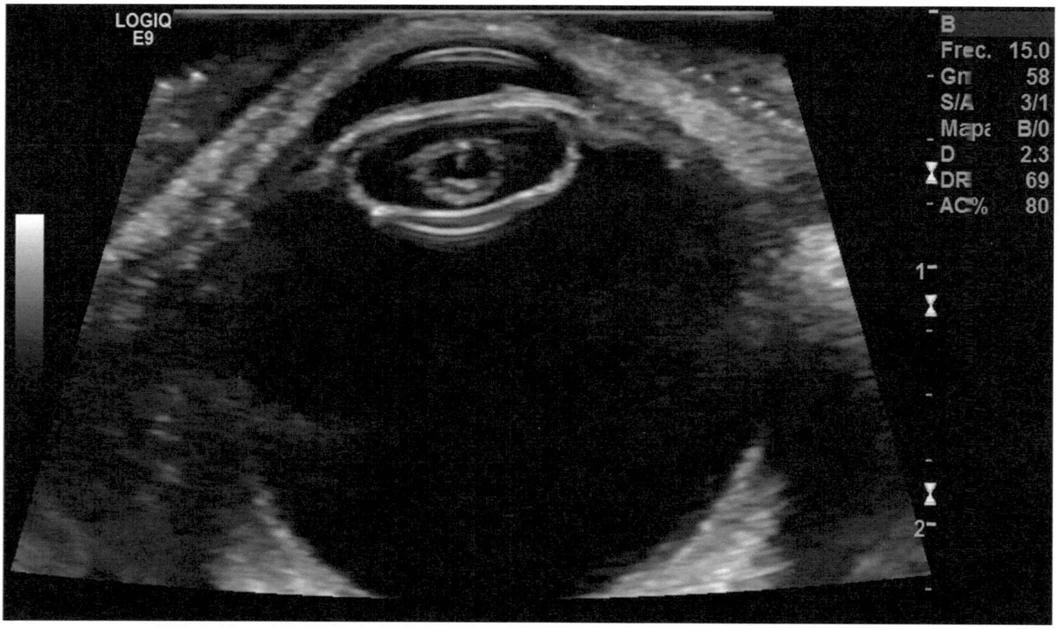

Figure 4: Sudden cataract with iris bombe.

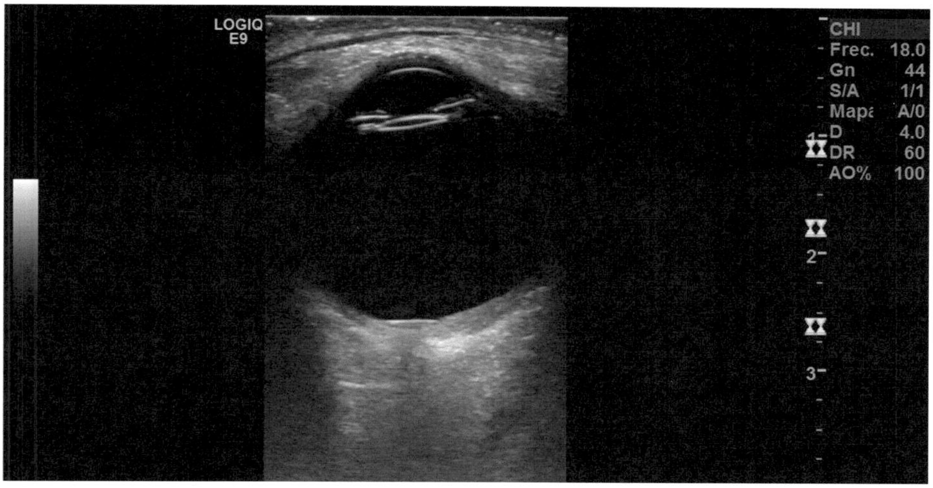

Figure 5: Intraocular lens.

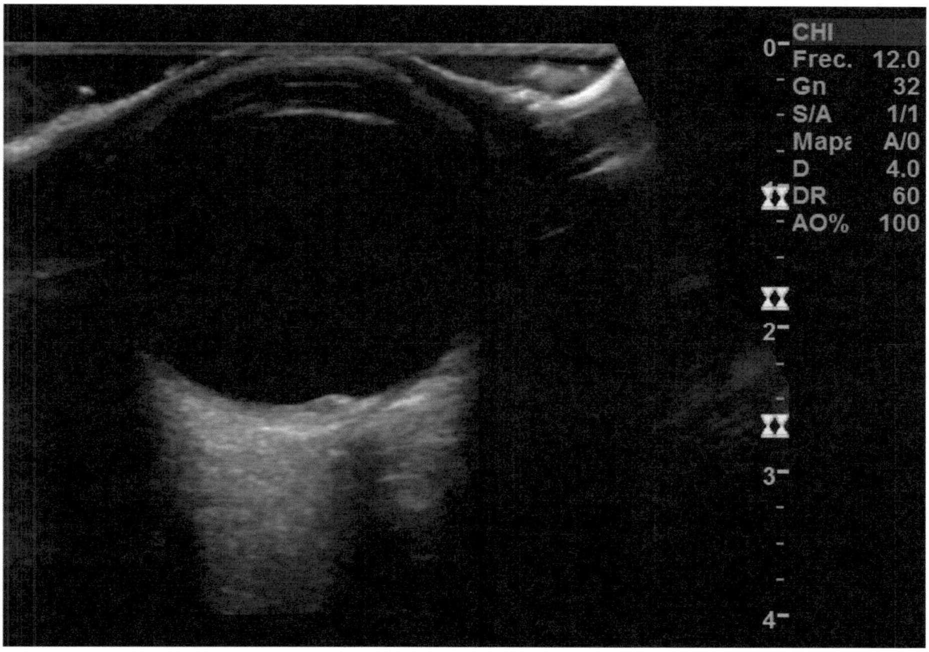

Figure 6: Normal vitreous body, echographic vitreous image.

that could lead to poor visualization of the retina. Often the retina requires echographic assessment in order to diagnose associated diseases which might be the cause of a retinal detachment in a patient with bleeding in the vitreous cavity. As a part of physiological processes, the vitreous body undergoes degeneration with age. This process is called syneresis, and is the result of degeneration of type II collagen fibers and the appearance of bags of liquefaction thereof inside. These changes result in the presence of hyper-echoic bands in the ultrasound, which moves jointly with the eye movements because these are not subjected to the wall of the ocular globe. Thereby, the ultrasound examination of the vitreous cavity is important as it allows to determine if vitreous body is anchored at the level of the entire retina, which would be its physiological position, or if it is detached from somewhere, what is called a posterior vitreous detachment. A number of times the posterior vitreous detachment is not complete, which means that we can see its lower part still attached to the inferior retina [4].

This fact becomes important for the prognosis of certain retinal pathologies, as in the case of proliferative diabetic retinopathy, in which the vitreous anchoring favors the retinal neovascularization grown. An important factor to consider in the ultrasonic scanning is that in certain situations the peripheral vitreous body adjacent to macular area undergoes liquefaction creating a liquid meniscus. This must not be confused with a posterior vitreous detachment, and the fact that it stays still despite the ocular globe movements helps us to distinguish each one of them. In the course of many vitrectomy surgeries, identifying this space is a very relevant aspect for the surgeon. In these situations some staining substances [as triamcinolone] are used to see the exact remains of the vitreous body attached to the retina.

The following important anatomical structure in the posterior segment is the retina. By means of ultrasound examination it is difficult to distinguish the retina from the other two adjacent structures [choroid and sclera], because all three have very small thickness and are hyper-echogenic. Retinal examination should be performed with transducers over 12 MHz, and must emphasize the exploration of the periphery of the retina, the macular area and the equatorial area [5-7]. One of the clearest indications for an echographic ophthalmic examination is to determinate the presence of retinal detachment if there are media opacities. The retina scan can be completed by using Color-Doppler ultrasound examination of the vessels derived from the central retinal artery and vein, which are in fact the only observable blood vessels, because the branches of these vessels are too small to be explored by color in this method [8-10]. The next layer is the posterior uvea or choroid. This is a vascular layer in its entirety which feeds oxygen to the retina and various substances necessary for its metabolism. The exploration of the choroid is important in case of inflammatory processes of the same, named uveitis, in which we observe the thickening of the whole layer. An abnormal thickening can also be observed in the presence of tumor pathologies.

Finally, the outer layer is the sclera, which is very hyper-echoic to ultrasound although with slight effect on ocular pathology. It's very important to evaluate the integrity of the sclera in the presence of ocular trauma, to rule out ocular globe perforations. The inflammatory condition of this layer called scleritis can also be assessed by ultrasound.

CONCLUDING REMARKS

The ocular echography with B-mode at 15 to 20 MHz ultrasounds, help us to observe ocular globe. The anterior segment is difficult to observe with current probes, but the posterior segment is clearly visualized with echography.

ACKNOWLEDGEMENTS

Declared None.

CONFLICT OF INTEREST

The authors confirm that this chapter contents have no conflict of interest.

REFERENCES

[1] Testut L, Latarjet A. Anatomía Humana. Capítulo IV Sentido de la vista. Editorial SALVAT SA. Barcelona 1980; 2555-729.

[2] Lorente-Ramos RM, Armán JA, Muñoz-Hernández A, *et al.* Use of the eye made easy: a comprehensive how-to review with ophthalmoscopic correlation. Radiographics. 2012; 32(5): 175-200.

[3] Ishikawa H, Schuman JS. Related Articles, Anterior segment imaging: ultrasound biomicroscopy.Ophthalmol Clin North Am. 2004; 17(1): 7-20.

[4] Herwig MC, Löffler KU, Wells JR, Grossniklaus HE. Clinico-pathological correlations: posterior compartment of the eye and orbit. Klin Monbl Augenheilkd. 2012; 229(7): 705-15.

[5] Braband K, Kerty E, Jakobsen JA. Contrast enhanced ultrasound Doppler examination of the retrobulbar arteries. Acta Radiol 2001; 42: 135.

[6] Harris A, Kagemann L, Cioffi G. Assessment of human ocular hemodynamics. Surv Ophthalmol 1998; 42: 509.

[7] Erickson SJ, Hendrix LE, Massaro BM, *et al.* Color-Doppler flow imaging of the normal and abnormal orbit. Radiology 1989; 173: 511.

[8] Lieb WE, Flaharty PM, Ho A, *et al.* Color-Doppler imaging of the eye and orbit. A synopsis of a 400-case experience. Acta Ophthalmol 1992; 204: 50.

[9] Baxter GM, Williamson TH. Color-Doppler flow imaging in central retinal vein occlusion: a new diagnostic technique? Radiology 1993; 187: 847.

[10] Braband K, Kerty E, Jakobsen JA. Contrast enhanced ultrasound Doppler examination of the retrobulbar arteries. Acta Radiol 2001; 42: 135.

Chapter 3: Ultrasound of the Anterior Segment

CHAPTER 3

Ultrasound of the Anterior Segment

Isabel Méndez-Marín* and Mónica Llagostera-Serra

Department of Ophthalmology, University Hospital Sant Joan, University Rovira and Virgili, Rovira & Virgili University, Pere Virgili Health Research Institute, IISPV, Reus, Spain

Abstract: The ultrasound in anterior segment has a great number of limitations, despite in patients with ocular cataract or with intraocular lens [IOL], has an important place. Furthermore is useful in patients with iris pathologies [iris tumours], or in patients with malignant glaucoma. The most important technique for anterior segment examination with ultrasounds is the ultrasonic biomicroscopy [UBM] technique, based on 35-50 MHz probes. In the next chapter we describe the UBM examination of anterior segment and its application in different pathologies as cornea diseases or glaucoma.

Keywords: Cornea, ultrasound biomicroscopy, corneal pathology, anterior segment, glaucoma, anterior globe injuries, biometry.

INTRODUCTION

1. Ultrasonic Biomicroscopy: Basics

The external and superficial location of the ocular globe and its cystic structure, together with the presence of the optical diaphragm [pupil] allow us to obtain precise images of their structures with different techniques: Optical coherence tomography [OCT], Magnetic resonance images [MRI], Scheimpflug-based corneal tomography, ultrasound and also by slit lamp examination.

Although optical methods offer high resolution and are easy to use, they cease to be useful in the presence of untransparent structures, both anatomical [sclera, iris] and pathological [hemorrhage, corneal scarring, dense cataracts].

Ultrasound images provide real-time, even in the presence of media opacities. The resolution of the ultrasound is increased with increasing frequency and bandwidth. The bandwidth refers to the range of frequencies present in a pulse of ultrasound. The higher the number of cycles by pulses, the lower the bandwidth and the

***Corresponding author Marc Baget-Bernaldiz:** Hospital Universitario Sant Joan, Avda. Doctor Josep Laporte 1 Reus, Spain; E-mail: imendez@grupsagessa.com

Pedro Romero-Aroca and Manuel Montero-Jaime (Eds.)

resolution. Therefore, for a high-resolution ultrasound image, there should be high frequencies and bandwidths. Ultrasonic examination of the anterior segment with conventional probes [7.5 to 10 MHz] allows to differentiate the structures, albeit with some difficulty, because the resolution of these transducers is not enough. The 10 MHz transducer using probes are targeted for the examination of the vitreous and retina [1-3]. Today we have high-frequency transducers [35-50 MHz] that allow us to perform a more comprehensive study of the anterior segment [ultrasound biomicroscopy] with a resolution of 40 mm or even less. These high frequency transducers are obtained from polyvinylidene fluoride membranes that can withstand up to 100 MHz frequencies without breakage, unlike zirconate titanate crystals. The ultrasonic biomicroscopy [UBM] is a technique based on ultrasound emission by a transducer which passes through the tissues and is then reflected to the receiver, thus providing information about their anatomy. The application of ultrasound technique to ophthalmology has been used for a long time, since the introduction of UBM which provided the opportunity to assess *in vivo* study of the ocular globe with a detail similar to histologic studies. The UBM is an immersion technique; it means a fluid medium is required between the probe and the surface of the ocular globe. The medium used may vary depending on circumstances; however, the technique always requires the patient to be in supine. Although there is no contact with the ocular surface, the examination must be performed under topical anesthesia.

2. Basic Instrumentation

- Field exploration: Using a transfer medium between the transducer and ocular globe requires to create a field of exploration that holds the immersion medium to achieve adequate resolution of the images. Different methods have been designed for this such as the scanning cups.

- Eyecup: A device made of methacrylate that is placed in contact with the ocular surface and has a central opening for the immersion medium and the transducer.

- This model allows scanning of the anterior and posterior chamber as well as the limbic area. By making the patient move the eye, we can also explore the pars plana and peripheral retina. The problem with this is that extreme eye movements lead to the loss of immersion medium and necessitating exploration to restart.

- Orbital Cup: This device has been designed to increase the field of exploration. It is a larger cup which lies on the upper and lower orbital rims, thus it is necessary to insert a speculum to keep the ocular surface exposed [3].

- It allows greater exposure of the field, and the wide central opening does not limit eye movements. In addition, the patient's eye movements allow a wide field: 15 mm in temporary limbo, 12 mm in nasal, 10 mm higher and 11 mm lower limb.

- Speculum: It is possible to perform an assessment without an eye cup or a surgical field by placing a speculum and the immersion medium. This method is fast, easy to use and offers a wide field of exploration. It is very useful in young children and uncooperative adults.

- Methylcellulose: It is the ideal immersion medium because it offers high quality images. It can be used at concentrations of 1 % or 2.5%. The latter, provides minimal losses in the fluid coupling medium, making easy the transmission of ultrasound and obtaining higher quality images. As a problem, it is expensive.

- Saline solution: It is the cheapest but offers greater difficulties. It can not be used in exploring without the eyecup. It is useful as a medium when used mixed with methylcellulose.

- Artificial tears: The high density artificial tears are only useful in assessments when we use a speculum. The probe tends to continuously sweep the tear and it has to be replaced.

- Corneal protection mechanisms: The use of fluid coupling medium and the stop security system of the probe if it touches the cornea are sufficient to protect the ocular cavity.

- Fixation Instruments: The cooperation of the patient in this exploration is mandatory. To maintain the patient, fixation is useful to place light dots on the ceiling of the examination room.

The new UBM systems are equipped with probes with fluid filled tips, allowing direct contact with the eye surface. These systems avoid using eyecups or orbital cups.

3. Anterior Segment Ultrasound Assessment

Images obtained with the 50 MHz transducer allow us to analyze the anterior structures of the ocular globe. The sharpness of the images depends on how perpendicular the ultrasound beam is, so as we move towards the periphery, the images lose quality. In any case, conventional transducers provide us useful images of the anterior segment, also easily obtained through the eyelids [4, 5].

4. Cornea

With conventional transducers, the eyelids and the conjunctiva surrounding the cornea result in a moderate echogenicity structure delimiting the anterior part of the anterior chamber. With higher resolution probes, cornea appears as a thin echogenic line convex, later limited by echogenic interface.

The exploration of the cornea by BMU allows us to appreciate the following structures in a normal scan:

- Epithelium and Bowman's membrane: Appear as two parallel hyper-reflective lines; in the periphery they tend to fuse.
- Stroma: Has low reflectivity structure and is very smooth.
- Descemet membrane-endothelium: a single hyper-reflective line that cannot be differentiated.
- Corneal-scleral Transition: It clearly appears as a gradual transition between the low reflectivity of the cornea and the hyper-reflectivity of the sclera.

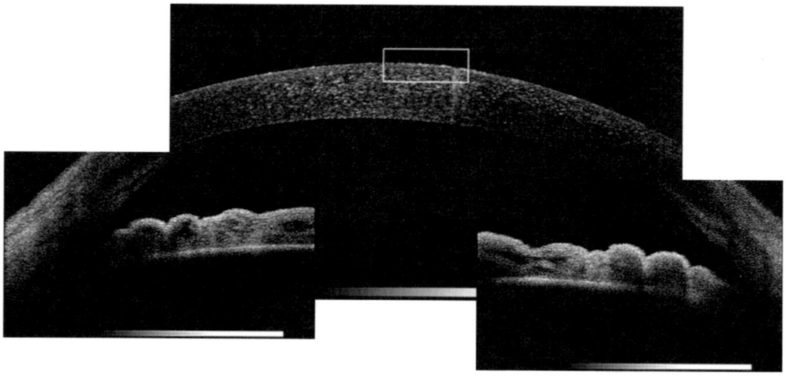

Figure 1: Photo-composition of the cornea and iris.

5. Anterior Chamber

It appears as an anechogenic area where the pupil appears as an anechoic disruption within the iris.

6. Iris

The iris usually appears as a rectilinear structure easily identifiable and sometimes has depressions in its front surface corresponding to the crypts (Fig. **1**). The pigmentary epithelium appears as a thick hyper-reflective line, unlike lower-middle echogenicity of the stroma, in which sometimes iris vessels can be found [6-8].

Conventional probes show the iris and ciliary body as less echogenic structures than the sclera, but do not offer the precise details as the UB (Fig. **2**).

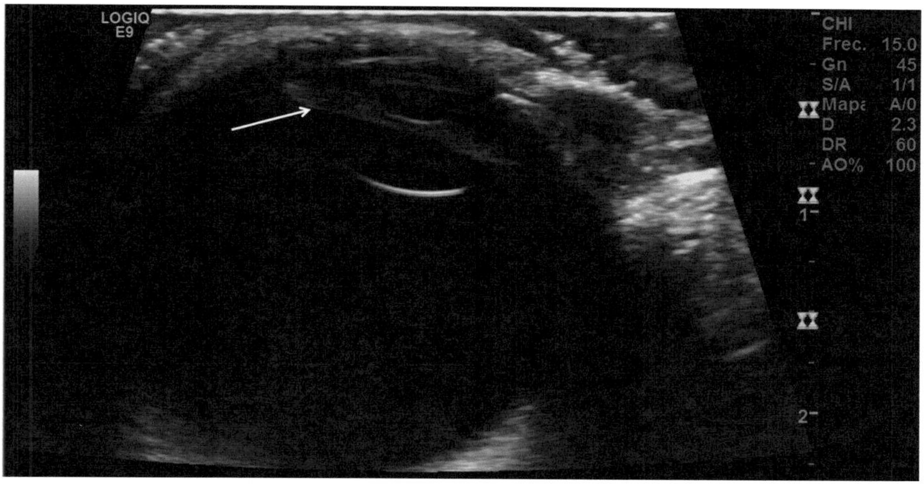

Figure 2: Normal iris, white arrow.

7. Posterior Chamber

Like the anterior chamber appears as an anechoic area, the posterior chamber can be observed in the peripheral of the globe.

8. Camerular Angle

It is the great discovery of the BMU. Browsing its greater or lesser extent, we must always make a reference to the scleral spur. Instead, Schwalbe's line is hardly distinguishable unless it is clearly hypertrophic. In conventional ultrasound, the rear camera appears as an anechoic area in close relation to the anterior lens surface.

9. Ciliary Body

The pars plicata has a reflectivity similar to iris stroma, showing clearly the ciliary processes in the cross sections. The pigment epithelium is clearly seen as a thick line being hyper-reflective.

The pars plana reflectivity shows the same apparent pigment epithelium. In this area one can see the inclusion of more posterior zonular fibers. These lines always appear as medium-high reflectivity that adopts the form of bundles.

10. Lens

As can be seen previously, the lens is visualized as an area of low reflectivity, except for the mature cataracts. The posterior capsule appears as a line of high reflectivity. With conventional transducers, the anterior surface is characterized as an area of higher reflectivity than the anterior surface of the iris, with the posterior surface being appreciated as a more defined with lower reflectivity.

11. Conjunctiva and Sclera

The high content of collagen of the sclera makes it an echogenic structure easily identifiable and distinguishable from the conjunctiva and uvea structures of lower middle echogenicity.

12. Peripheral Retina and Choroid

These structures experience difficulty in exploring the orbital except with a glass or speculum. The most accessible area is the temporal retina. The choroid appears as a low echogenic area below the ciliary body, between two hyper reflective lines: complex sclera and retina-retinal pigment epithelium [RPE]. In contrast, the broader field of conventional transducers allows us to differentiate the increased echogenicity of the sclera and its intimate relationship with the ciliary body.

OCULAR PATHOLOGY

1. Pathology of the Cornea

Initially, one might think that there are not advantages in using the UBM because the cornea is an easily assessable structure by optical biomicroscopy. However, in cases of loss of corneal transparency, the UBM provides us a valuable information that is not available by exploring the anterior segment structures. In cases of corneal edema, the epithelium becomes thick and irregular, which can be seen as a thickness space between the two hyperreflective lines formed by the epithelium and the Bowman membrane. When the edema affects the corneal stroma, we can observe the thickening and the homogeneous increase of echogenicity due to the accumulation of fluid between the stromal lamellae. Once the edema is resolved, resulting leukoma is shown as an increase in reflectivity that may be diffused or localized [9-11]. With a conventional transducer we are able to see the presence of corneal thickening and corneal endothelium integrity. The assessment of the endothelium and Descemet's membrane in edematous corneas can guide us to the origin of the edema, *i.e.*, guttae cornea in Fuch's distrophy [12, 13], or Descemet dehiscence (Fig. **3**).

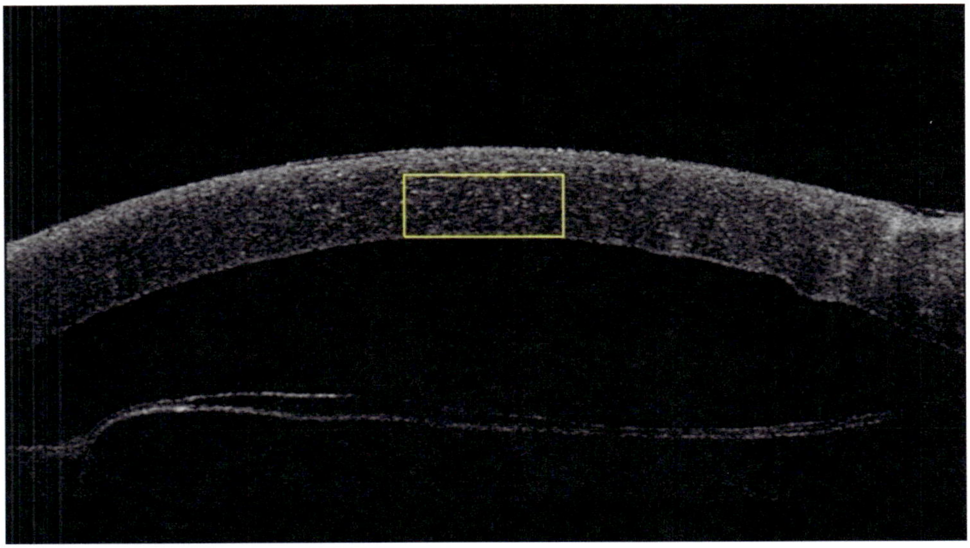

Figure 3: The double hyper-reflective line in anterior chamber is the Descemet, in a case of dehiscence.

2. Crystalline Lens and Intraocular Lens

As mentioned above, the UBM and the conventional 10 to 18 MHz echography offer poor quality images behind the crystalline lens but it is important to study the location and position of the intraocular lens [IOL]. Preoperative evaluation may be important to detect cases of cysts of iris or ciliary body, plateau iris, posterior and anterior synechiae and lens subluxation. The presence of nuclear and cortical cataracts is shown as areas of high internal reflectivity.

Echogenicity of intraocular lenses varies depending on the material they are made of. PMMA and hydrophilic lenses show two hyperechoic lines corresponding to the anterior and posterior superficies, and a posterior acoustic shadowing. Silicone lenses do not allow the passage of ultrasound and thus show a hyperreflective line followed by a hyporeflective zone. Hydrogel lenses look similar to the silicone lenses, but with less posterior attenuation. In contrast, collagen lenses produce very little attenuation and enable posterior structures to be observed easily, as in the phakic lenses.

The UBM and conventional 10 to 18 MHz echographies allow us to appreciate luxations of intraocular lenses that are not observable by slit lamp examination (Fig. **4**). In anterior chamber lenses we can observe malposition of the haptics or if there is contact with the iris or endothelium. In posterior chamber lenses we can see if the haptics are in the bag or sulcus and in the latter case, check whether or not there is contact with the iris. Furthermore, it is very interesting to know the position of the haptics in the sutured lens cases, and their relationship with the surrounding tissues.

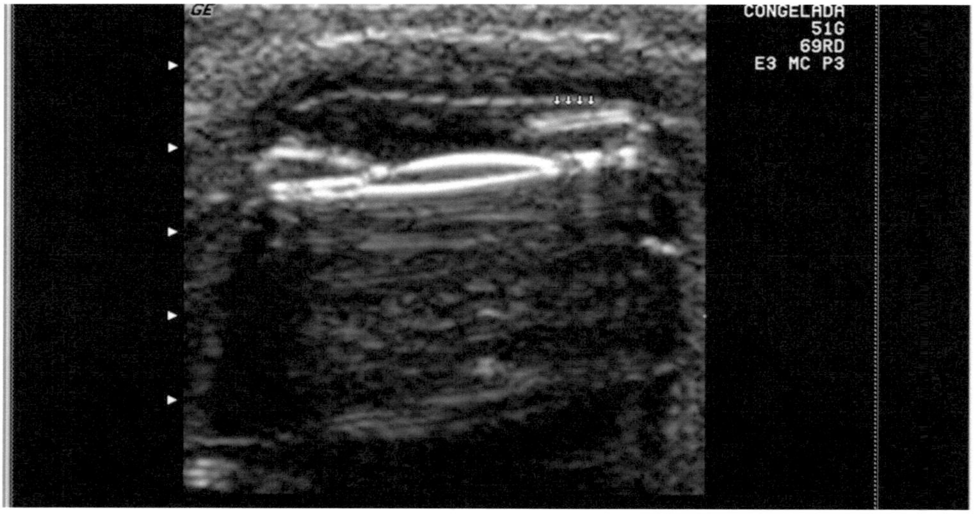

Figure 4: Subluxation of IOL, the left IOL haptic is closely to iris than right haptic, white arrows indicate the right iris

3. Glaucoma

The UBM cannot discriminate the fine iris angle structures and thus it is not superior to the gonioscopic observation of the angle structures, but it can provide information concerning the relationship between the body of the iris and ciliary processes [14-16]. The importance of ultrasound imaging is stressed in the evaluation of the effectiveness of glaucoma surgical procedures.

The lack of differentiation of the fine structures has led some authors to define parameters used to determine the morphological characteristics of the angle and its correlation with scanning classifications based on gonioscopy. Other authors propose angle assessment by Angle Opening Distance [ODA] to 250 mm and 500 mm. ODA 250 is calculated by drawing a line from a point scleral spur in the endothelium of the same 250 mm, and then drawing a perpendicular to the endothelium from that point to the anterior surface of the iris.

- Glaucoma: Pathogenetic aspects

  In open angle glaucoma, the UBM is useful to differentiate many pathogenic aspects. In primary glaucoma one can only assess the presence of an open angle; in pseudoexfoliative syndrome it is possible to observe the presence of the material deposited on the pupillary area and in several structures of the anterior and posterior chamber. In the pigment dispersion syndrome, much more information could be provided by this technique. The UBM has allowed us to distinguish two pathogenic types of pigmentary glaucoma: a group in which the iris concavity is increased causing continuous friction with the ciliary processes and zonular ligaments and a second group in which the slit lamp assessment seems normal. Dynamic UBM has shown that during the crystalline lens accommodation process in these eyes, there is a displacement behind the insertion of the iris thus leading to an increase in contact between the iris and the ciliary body. In the presence of traumatic glaucoma, the UBM allows us to appreciate more easily the presence of iridodialysis or cyclodialysis which could be barely observable by gonioscopy assessment and is especially useful in cases when there is blood or there are inflammatory membranes on the anterior chamber. In closed-angle glaucoma, UBM gives a clear picture: iris-crystalline anterior diaphragm, narrowing of the anterior chamber and the entrance of the anterior chamber angle. In plateau-iris glaucoma, the use of the UBM has helped to define the etiology of this condition. Pavlin [5-7] appreciated that the ciliary processes are rotated above and contact the rear surface of the iris causing its typical plateau configuration. In these patients, the UBM has shown that the iridotomy does not change the position of the ciliary processes and therefore does not change the angle closure. As we can see, the UBM is a technique that allows knowledge of the position angle and anatomic variations of the iris and ciliary body [17-21].

- Glaucoma: Surgical features

The UBM has helped determine the functional mechanisms of many surgical procedures and how these procedures reduce the intraocular pressure. Until recently, trabeculectomy has been the surgical technique of choice in the treatment of open-angle glaucoma. Trabeculectomy may lower IOP by the following mechanisms: (a) Pass of aqueous humor into Schlemm's canal by side gaps which have remained open after removing the trabeculum in the trabeculectomy. This aspect has not been tested by the UBM. (b) Pass of aqueous humor through the internal ostium into intrascleral space. Once there, it can filter the aqueous humor into the vessels. In these cases the UBM allows us to appreciate an anechoic space which is an indicator of the intrascleral filtration through internal ostium.

ANTERIOR SEGMENT TUMORS

Conventional echography cannot detect lesions less than 0.8 mm or 3 mm lower elevations. The UBM uses high frequencies to detect small lesions in the anterior segment with a high resolution.

1. Iris Tumors

The most common tumors of the iris are derived from melanocytes. The benign and malignant tumors derived from epithelial cells are very uncommon. The basic difference between a freckle and nevus is that macroscopically, a freckle respects and maintains the crypts and iris morphology; even in the UBM a freckle shows no findings. Nevi are detected as an increase in thickness of the iris, but with a homogeneous internal reflectivity without changing the internal structure. Iris melanomas are rare and appear after fourth decade of life. Circumscribed melanomas may look like nevi but some details can lead us toward their malignancy. The UBM can detect the breakdown of the iris and the presence of feeder vessels in the tumor and invasion of surrounding structures.

2. Ciliary Body Tumors

Melanoma is the most common tumor of the ciliary body. It has a high anterior reflectivity, with a lack of penetration of the echoes. The origin of the melanoma is difficult to determine. Normally, it is considered that the original structure is the one in which the tumor is most extended. Of course, the UBM provides useful information concerning tumor growth and compression and displacement of adjacent structures.

INJURIES OF ANTERIOR SEGMENT

The lesions in the anterior segment can be observed by UBM and in cases of media opacity: corneal edema, hyphema, and subconjunctival hemorrhages can help us to see the damaged structures. By using UBM we can observe the presence of iridodialysis, anterior capsule rupture, lens dislocation, cyclodialysis, zonular defects, angle recession and intraocular foreign bodies. Being a non-contact technique, it may be used in perforating trauma with minimal compression of the structures. In these situations the UBM is very important in accurate diagnosis and treatment planning.

CONCLUDING REMARKS

The future of the UBM passes through obtaining new annular array transducers [*i.e.*, piezoelectric concentric rings allowing for the emission of higher frequencies]. In the coming years the emergence of a combined ultrasound and optical system, called photo-acoustic image may be possible. This technique consists of the emission of nanosecond optical pulses, causing themoelastic expansion of tissues as a result of light absorption. This will allow us photoacoustic imaging of specific molecules such as hemoglobin [images of the microvasculature] or melanin [located in uvea and tumors].

The anterior segment ultrasound examination requires high ultrasound resolution and only ultrasonic biomicroscopy [UBM] technique, based on 35-50 MHz probes, permitting to examine the cornea, anterior chamber and lens structures. The uses of conventional ultrasound at 15 to 20 MHz permit us to observe the iris structure, and lens or the intraocular lens position.

ACKNOWLEDGEMENTS

Declared None.

CONFLICT OF INTEREST

The authors confirm that this chapter contents have no conflict of interest.

REFERENCES

[1] Silverman R. High-resolution ultrasound imaging of the eye – a review. Clin Expert Ophthalmol 2009; 37(1): 54-67.

[2] Garcia-Feijoo J, Martín-Carbajo M, Benitez del Castillo JM, García-Sánchez J. Orbital cup: A device to facilitate ultrasound biomicroscopic examination of pars plana and peripheral retina. Arch Ophthalmol 1997; 115: 1475-76.

[3] Tello C, Liebmann J, Rich R. An improved coupling médium for ultrasound biomicroscopy. Ophthalmic Surg 1994; 25: 410-11.

[4] Ursea R, Silverman RH. Anterior-segment imaging for assessment of glaucoma. Expert Rev Ophthalmol 2010 1; 5(1): 59-74.

[5] Pavlin CJ, Harasiewicz K, Foster FS. Ultrasound biomicroscopy of anterior structures in normal and glaucomatous eyes. Am J Ophthalmol 1992; 113: 381-9.

[6] Pavlin CJ, Ritch R, Sherar MD, *et al.* Ultrasound biomicroscopy in plateau iris syndrome. Am Ophthalmol 1992; 113: 390-5.

[7] Wand M, Pavlin CJ, Foster FS. Plateau iris syndrome ultrasound biomicroscopy and histologic study. Ophthalmic Surgery 1993; 2: 129-131.

[8] Branco Ramos JL. Clinical and resarch applications of anterior segmento optical coherence tomography – a review. Clin Experiment Ophthalmol 2009; 397(1): 81-9.

[9] Yuen LH . Biometry of the cornea and anterior chamber in Chinese eyes: an anterior segment optical coherence tomography study. Invest Ophthalmol & Visc Scien. July 2010, 51(7): 3433-40. .

[10] Prisant O, Calderon N, Chastang P *et al.* Reliability of pachimetric measurements using Orbscan after excimer refractive surgery. Ophthalmology 2003; 110(3): 511-5.

[11] Khurana RN, Li Y, Tang M *et al.* High-speed optical coherence tomography of corneal opacities. Ophthalmology 2007; 114(7): 1278-85.

[12] Maldonado *et al.* Optical Coherence Tomography Evaluation of the corneal cap and estromal bed features after Laser In Situ Keratomileusis for High Myopia and Astigmatism. Opthalmology 2000; 107: 81-8.

[13] Asrani S, Sarunic M, Santiago C, *et al.* Detailed visualization of the anterior segment using Fourier-Domain Optical Coherence Tomography. Arch Ophthalmol 2008; 126(6): 765-71.

[14] Christopher KS *et al.* Visualization of anterior chamber angle dynamics using optical coherence tomography. Ophthalmology 2005; 112: 980-4.

[15] Wirbelauer C, Karandish A, Haberle H, *et al.* Noncontact goniometry with optical coherence tomography. Arch Ophthalmol 2005; 123: 179-5.

[16] Sakata LM. Assesment of the sclera spur in anterior segment optical coherence tomography images. Arch Ophthalmol 2008; 126: 181-5.

[17] Sakata LM, Raghavan L, Friedman DS *et al.* Comparison of gonioscopy and anterior segment ocular coherence tomography in detecting angle closure in different quadrants of the anterior chamber angle. Ophthalmology 2008; 115: 769-74. .

[18] Geerling G, Muller M, Winter C *et al.* Intraoperative 2-dimensional optical coherence tomography as a new tool for anterior segment surgery. Arch Ophthalmol 2005; 123(2): 253-7.

[19] Wong H, Lim M Friedman DS *et al.* High-Definition optical coherence tomography imaging of the iridocorneal angle of the eye. Arch Ophthalmol 2009; 127: 256-60.

[20] Li Y, Tang M, Zhang X. Pachymetric mapping with Fourier-Domain Optical Coherence Tomography. J Cataract Refract Surg 2010; 36(5): 826-31.

[21] Silverman RH, Kong F, Chen YC *et al.* High-Resolution Photoacoustic imaging of ocular tissues. Ultrasound Med Biol 2010; 36(5): 733-42.

CHAPTER 4

Ultrasound in the Posterior Segment

Pedro Romero-Aroca[1,*], Manuel Montero-Jaime[2,*], Marc Baget-Bernaldiz[1] and Javier Reyes-Torres[1]

[1]Department of Ophthalmology, [2]Department of Radiology, University Hospital Sant Joan, Rovira & Virgili University, Pere Virgili Health Research Institute, IISPV, Reus, Spain

Abstract: The ultrasound in posterior segment pathologies is the gold standard examination technique in cases of media opacities, when a cataract or vitreous hemorrhage exists. The first technique used to visualize the posterior segment is the echography. The ultrasound examination is fundamental in retina pathologies as retinal detachment in patients with cataracts. Its importance has been increased with the introduction of color Doppler echography which helps us in vasculophaties as arterial or venous occlusions or in patients with diabetic retinopathy. Furthermore, echography is useful in postoperative vitreous-retina patients, to detect new retinal detachments or peripheral new vessels growth in cases of recidivant hemorrhages.

Keywords: Vitreous echography, retina echography, choroid echography, scleral ultrasound, retinal detachment, vitreous hemorrhage, diabetic retinopathy, uveitis echography.

INTRODUCTION

The application of ultrasound in ocular pathology is indeed important, in the posterior segment diseases of the eye where it has its maximum indication. The examination of the vitreous, retina, and choroid can be easily performed by ophthalmoscopy if the medium of the eye is transparent. Even certain exploration techniques as fluorescein angiography and computed tomography [CT] are highly useful and necessary for the diagnosis of pathological entities affecting the posterior segment [1], but all these techniques require an excellent visualization of this. In many occasions, unfortunately, there is no transparency in the medium of the eye as in cases of existing corneal opacities, cataracts, or vitreous opacities; in all these cases, ultrasound has a high diagnostic utility. On the other hand,

***Corresponding author Manuel Montero-Jaime:** Hospital Universitario Sant Joan, Avda. Doctor Josep Laporte 1 Reus, Spain; E-mail: mmontero@grupsagessa.com
Pedro Romero Aroca: Hospital Universitario Sant Joan, Avda. Doctor Josep Laporte 1 Reus, Spain; E-mail: pormero@grupsagessa.com

Pedro Romero-Aroca and Manuel Montero-Jaime (Eds.)

whether the medium of the eye is transparent, the ultrasound provides basic information for the correct diagnosis of certain pathologies, and thus it clearly differentiates between a serous detachment and a hemorrhagic choroidal detachment. In other entities such as the melanoma choroid, the observed signs on ultrasound aid to the correct diagnosis of this tumor [2].

VITREOUS PATHOLOGY

The vitreous is an anechoic structure that is anteriorly limited with the lens, which is housed within the zonules and the ciliary body in the hyaloid fossa; and it is weakly attached to the retina at its posterior lateral side. It is covered by the vitreous membrane, or hyaloid, which is not normally identified on ultrasound in normal conditions. Between the hyaloid and the sensory retina is the virtual subhyaloid space. During the embryologic development, the hyaloid canal, or Cloquet's canal exists with the hyaloid artery that feeds the lens [3]. This is commonly denominated as primary vitreous; its persistence is due to leukocoria. It represents two-thirds of the ocular volume due to being constituted by a network of collagen fibers, water, glycoproteins and hyaluronic acid. This composition determines, before the aggressions, a prevailing fibroproliferative type of response with the consequent risk of traction on the sensory retina. Changes occur with age, which basically are the thickening and decreased volume.

The study of the vitreous using 10 MHz probes is successful, but if we want to observe injuries near of the posterior pole, by increasing its resolution, we will have to increase the power of the probe from 10 MHz to 20 MHz maximum [4]. For the vitreous cavity, the ultrasonic study on the interface between vitreous and retina, especially the determination of the posterior hyaloid, is difficult to be explored with 10 MHz, or even 20 MHz. The acoustic impedance difference of 10 MHz between the vitreous and the orbit may lead to the formation of a false echogenic artifact between the vitreous and the posterior pole. This artifact, result of the reverberation, can seriously make the analysis of the vitreomacular interface difficult as well the appreciation of the posterior hyaloid situation in front of the macular region; since with a reduced gain, the hyaloid is not reflective enough to be displayed; and if the gain is at its peak, it can be lost in the noise emitted by the artifacts. If we increase the frequency to values higher than 10 MHz and close to 20 MHz, we need to increase the gain in order to detect the existing fine vitreous structures in front of the posterior pole, which can be lost amid the overall background noise of the image [5].

1. Concept of Gain in the Study of the Vitreous

In ultrasound studies of the vitreous, the gain of the ultrasound beam and the dynamic exploration is particularly important. With the increase in the gain, we can identify the pathological situations and the physiological changes associated with aging. As the healthy vitreous is anechogenic, it is difficult to explore it using ultrasound; in order to solve this, we have to resort to the study by a maximum gain of ultrasound that complicates, however, the display of other structures of the eye or of the orbit. On the contrary, the study using standard gain allows us to quantify the possible vitreous membranes, and the possible adhesions between vitreous and retina (Fig. **1**).

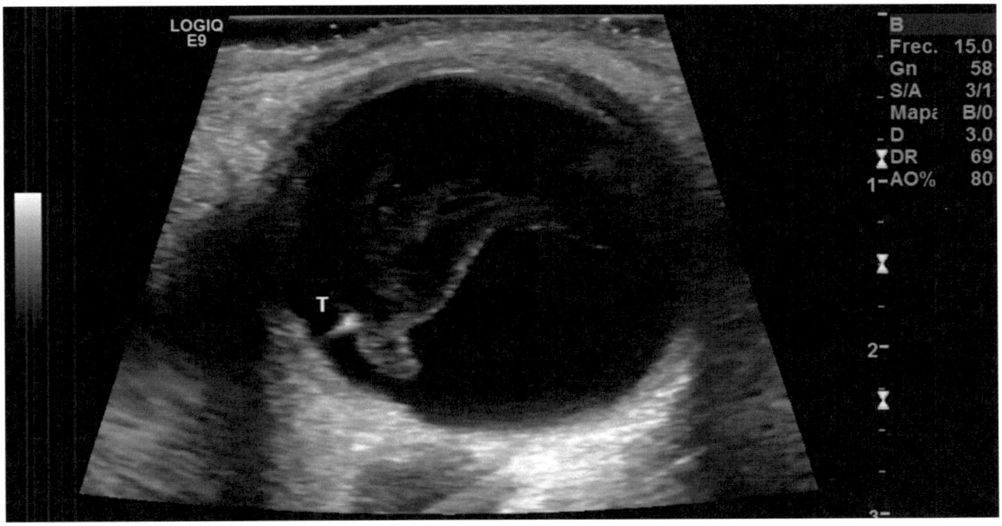

Figure 1: Vitreous-retina adhesion, in a case of posterior vitreous detachment. Letter T indicate the vitreous-retinal attachment.

2. Concept of Dynamic Ultrasound

The realization of a dynamic or kinetic study is the basic matter in the study of the vitreous., In the realization of a dynamic study, the patient is asked to make lateral and vertical movements of the ocular globe, since the eye movements move the vitreous gel and their possible components; it allows us not only to identify membranes, hemorrhage, areas vitreous liquefaction and vitreous detachment, but we will also rate their relationship with the retina, and it will be useful in the differential diagnosis with other pathologies [5]. The ultrasound greatly assists the diagnosis in any pathology, as is in the case of vitreous opacities. Precisely, it is in these cases where other exploration techniques of fundus examination do not provide us with relevant information, where the ocular echography will give us information about the state of the retina, and the possible opacity's origin that we observe, and thus the presence of a vitreous hemorrhage makes the visualization of the fundus of the eye difficult, but ultrasound helps to diagnose a retinal detachment or a proliferative diabetic retinopathy. The origin of the opacities in the vitreous may be by hemorrhagic, inflammatory [posterior uveitis], degenerative (Fig. **2**), or secondary to other pathologies [myopia, asteroid hyalosis or amyloidosis].

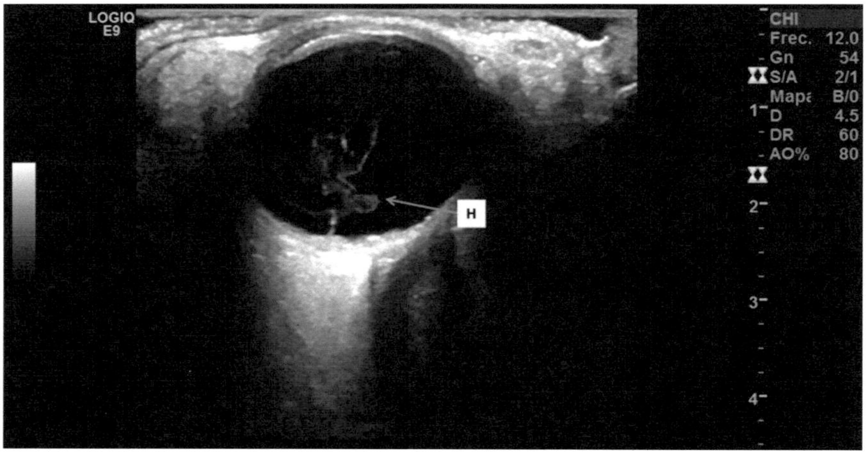

Figure 2: Posterior vitreous detachment, with hialoides collapse (H)

3. Hemorrhage in Vitreous

Hemorrhage in vitreous is the first indication of ultrasound usage in ocular pathology; its origin may be secondary to:

- Rhegmatogenous or tractional retinal detachment.
- Vitreous detachment that has torn retinal vessels or it has produced a tear in the retina.
- Presence of a diabetic retinopathy that may be or not proliferative.
- Presence of a tumor in the retina or the choroid.
- Presence of a macular degeneration associated to age which produces a hemorrhage, not only in the subretinal space, but crosses to the vitreous cavity.

Besides providing information about its origin, the information provided about the extent of the hemorrhage is important, if it occupies the entire vitreous cavity, or if only limits itself to the retrohyaloid space or otherwise locates itself in the vitreous but without filling the space of the retrohyaloid space. We must consider that if the hemorrhage is located exclusively in the retrohyaloid space, it is an indication for vitreous surgery because of the retinal toxicity that its presence has. Besides, the ultrasound is highly useful because its application in real time gives us information about its movement, and if it is anchored at some point on the retina, it could lead to traction, retinal tears, or detachment in those areas (Fig. **3**).

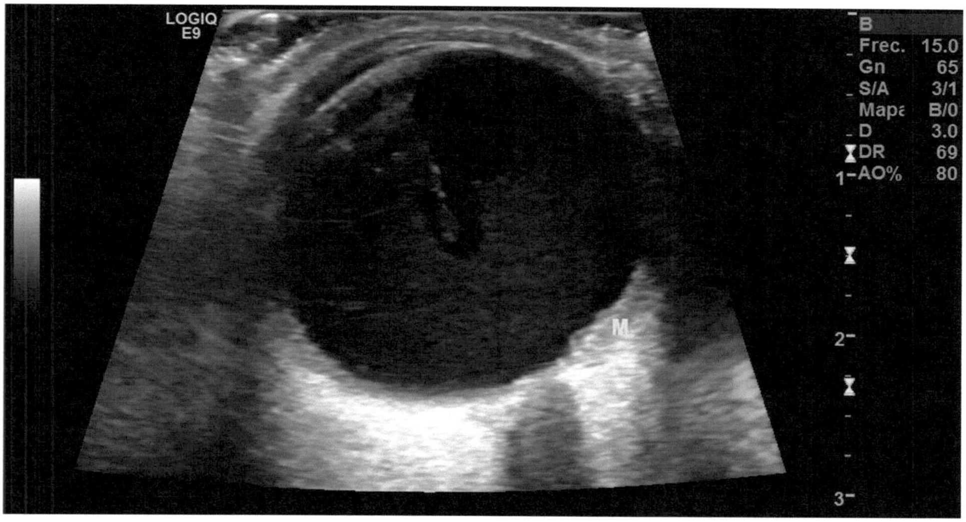

Figure 3: Vitreous hemorrhage, a dense ultrasound image fills the vitreous.

4. Hemorrhages in Vitreous Gel

The echographic appearance varies in function of the amount and length of hemorrhage. Mild hemorrhages determine a normal exploration with minimal echoes in the posterior pole. More substantial acute hemorrhages are seen as floating echoes that move freely along the eye movements. In the subacute chronic hemorrhages, clots are formed, identified as irregularities of heterogeneous echo-structure. Subsequently, tracts or membranes appear (Fig. **3**). These membranes usually show a wavy aspect, are moderately echogenic, free or attached on one end of the eye's periphery. Over time, they can simulate a mainly peripheral retinal detachment. The differentiating criteria are the minor echogenicity of the membranes and the identification of a front bracketing to the ora serrata. If the membrane is highly echogenic, it shows the level of the anchoring in the disc, and it is posterior to the ora serrata, the probability of a DR is higher. We can also demonstrate the presence of retinal vascularization with a Color-Doppler study [6, 7]. If the hemorrhage lasts for weeks or months in the vitreous cavity [hemorrhage that clinically we defined as organized], it significantly increases its hyperreflectivity on ultrasound, complicating its differentiation regarding the inflammatory origin opacities.

5. Retrohyaloid Hemorrhage

In this case we observed a thin echogenic band, more or less wavy, that corresponds to the hyaloid and echoes in the retrohyaloid space, which is not often organized in membranes. This is because the blood does not clot itself in that space by not allowing the arising of more or less dense areas. If the amount of blood count is significant, a level can be observed in the retrohyaloid space (Fig. 4). As in the previous case, it is important to conduct a kinetics ultrasound in order to give us information about the displacement of the hemorrhage when moving the ocular globe [8], and even, you can ask the patient to lift his head showing inferior displacement of the hemorrhage.

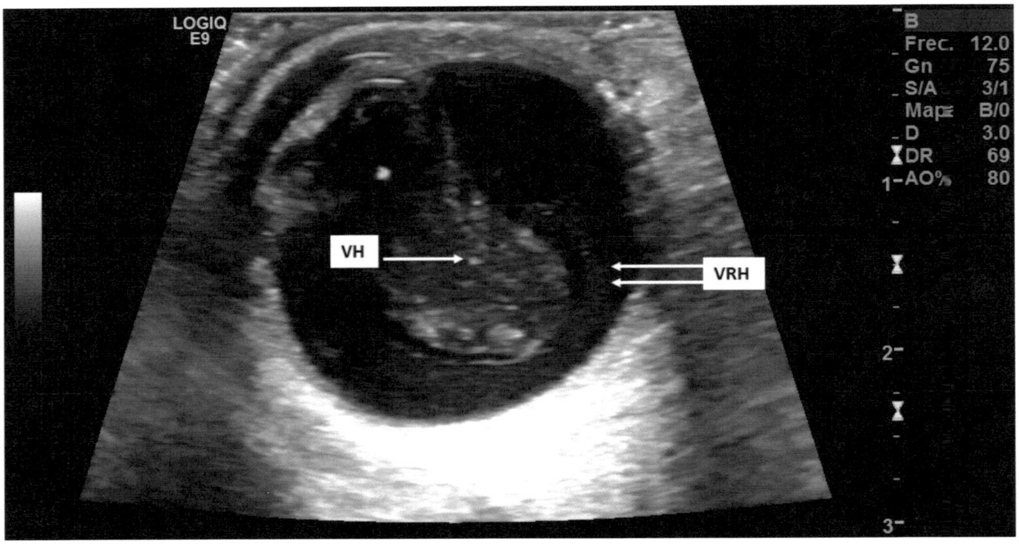

Figure 4: Vitreous-retinal hemorrhage [VH, one arrow] with retro-hyaloid hemorrhage [VRH, two arrows].

6. Hemorrhage in Vitrectomized Patients

A special feature of the blood in the cavity of a vitrectomized patient is that this does not clot. When conducting the ultrasound, we can observe the presence of vitreous gel traces, usually located in the most anterior part of the vitreous cavity seen as "tails" of the vitreous gel that move on kinetic echography (Fig. **5**).

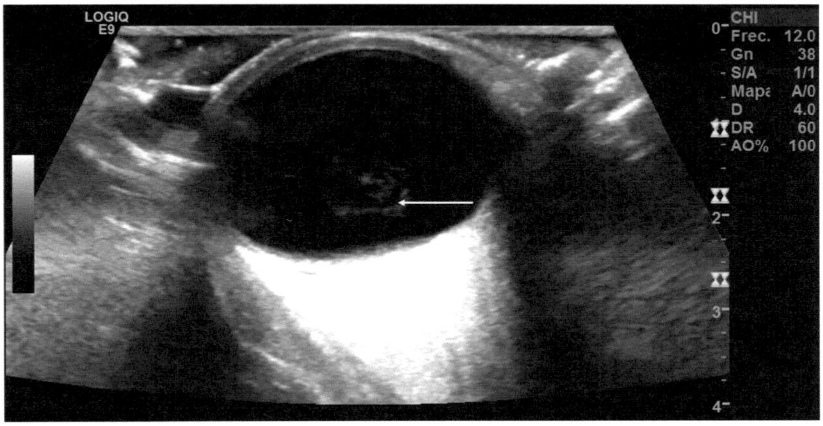

Figure 5: Vitreous gel traces, seen as "tails" of the vitreous gel that move on kinetic ultrasonography (white arrow), this is a normal senescent finding of the vitreous.

7. Inflammatory Opacities

The study of the inflamed vitreous by ultrasonic probes of 10 or 20 MHz will not give us much information about the number of cells or the inflammation amount present in the vitreous, but we do need more studies on them. Inflammatory opacities can be secondary to:

- Endo-ocular postoperative infections such as the endophthalmitis.
- Posterior uveitis with or without infectious origin.
- Panophthalmitis with the involvement of anterior and posterior segment.

While the ultrasound does not give us the origin of the opacity, it allows us to detect the presence of associated pathology such as tractional or exudative detachment; in the latter case, it must be differentiated, mainly, from a rhegmatogenous detachment. In all these cases ultrasound gives us information about the extent of the opacities inside the vitreous cavity, to be useful for example in cases of intermediate uveitis, in which the most posterior vitreous is not affected. The echographic patterns of inflammatory opacities in the vitreous have a limited mobility, which we can see in real-time ultrasound by observing the scarce shifting of the opacified vitreous in its cavity.

Vitreous Degenerations

Basically, the degeneration of the vitreous can be:

- Myopia
- Asteroid hyalosis
- Synchysis scintillans
- Amyloidosis

In these cases, the observed opacities in the vitreous are not uniform, particularly in the case of asteroid hyalosis; the particles are formed by calcium soaps which are highly hyper reflective on ultrasound (Figs. **6**, **7**). In general, on all the cases above, we can see hyper reflective echoes, in the ultrasound, scattered in the vitreous cavity with a homogeneous distribution, with very high mobility; in the case of being associated with posterior vitreous detachment, we can see that the echoes are confined to the vitreous leaving the retrohyaloid space free. Special case may be the myopic patient, in which one can observe an increase in the axial length between cornea and retina, especially in high myopia; in these cases one can observe the presence of vitreous detachment at an early age, especially in its part most posterior, with hyper reflective vitreous condensations in the ultrasound inside the vitreous gel and the hyaloid. Several researches have shown a good correlation between the ultrasound observations and the biomicroscopic study of the vitreous cavity [9-12]. Ultrasound, also, can provide information about the asteroid hyalosis origin; this may be secondary to a former retinal detachment or a proliferative diabetic retinopathy.

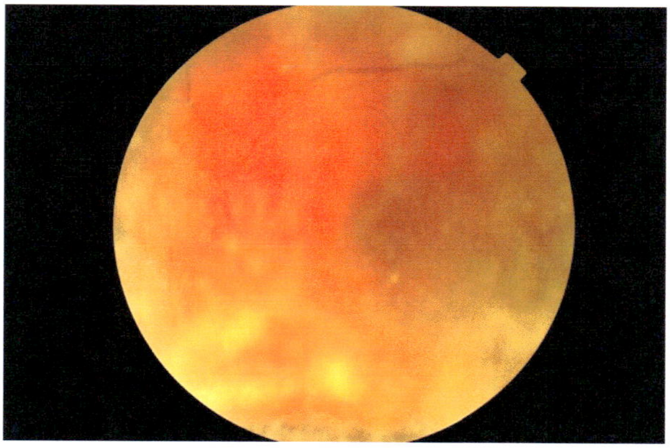

Figure 6: Asteroid Hyalosis [yellow opacities in the vitreous], is a degeneration of the vitreous

VASCULAR PATHOLOGY OF THE RETINA

Retinal vascular retinopathies include diabetic retinopathy and secondary to arterial hypertension, the venous and arterial occlusions, and could involve the inflammatory vascular diseases such as vasculitis. The information provided by ultrasound in these conditions can be very useful for its handling, since they often go with a hemorrhage in the vitreous, which hinders their correct diagnosis.

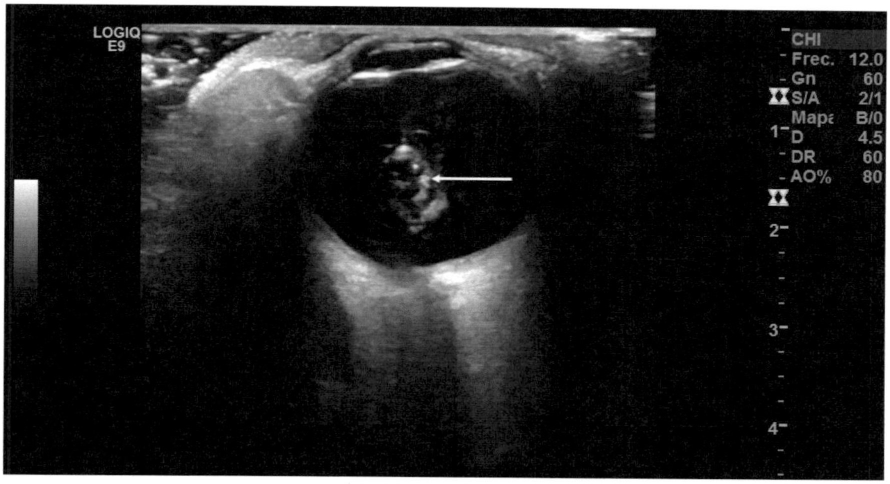

Figure 7: Asteroid Hyalosis [white arrow], is a degeneration of the vitreous.

1. Diabetic Retinopathy

In this condition, the ultrasound is useful to determine several entities that appear during the development of retinal diabetic microangiopathy, and its implementation is useful for:

- To observe the presence of posterior vitreous detachment, and to determine its scope.
- To determine the presence of posterior vitreoschisis.
- To establish the presence of vitreous hemorrhage and its location
- To observe the existence of neovascular proliferations in the retina
- To observe the presence of tractional retinal detachment.
- Study of the diabetic macular edema.

2. Ultrasound Findings

Its study is important because many complications of diabetic retinopathy include the involvement of the vitreous. During ultrasound, it the presence, or absence, of vitreous detachment of its retinal anchors demands attention. Usually the detachment occurs, at first, in the temporal periphery extending to the rest of the vitreous (Fig. **2**). It is important to determine if there are adhesions in the most posterior part of the retina, at the level of the pupil or the macula, as the former can be a source of retinal vitreous proliferations, and the latter can lead to tractions of the macular area. We must not forget that the presence of the hemorrhage in the vitreous may be largely caused within the context of diabetic retinopathy, referring to the previous chapter for its exploration. Within the study of the diabetic vitreous it is important to notice the vitreous cortex in front of the macular area; in this area, it often appears what is called vitreoschisis, which is the appearance of an area without vitreous gel [liquefaction of the vitreous], and which in its meniscus shape, is frequently confused with the presence of posterior vitreous detachment (Fig. **8**), but the hyaloid actually remains adhered to the retina in this area by being of common origin of fibrovascular diabetic proliferations [26]. This cavity appears even in the seventeen percent of patients with diabetic retinopathy. Echographically, the posterior edge of the cavity is less echogenic than the vitreous hyaloid; sometimes though, this distinction is not possible. Actually, the presence of vitreoschisis causes disparity between ultrasound findings and surgical findings in many cases [13].

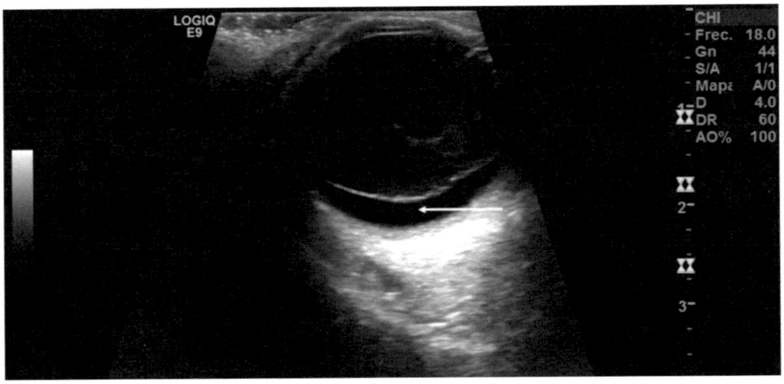

Figure 8: Cortical vitreous pocket, vitreosquisis [white arrow].

3. Diabetic Vitreous Hemorrhage

The ultrasound findings are the same as those described in the previous section; and to those, we refer to the reader to just emphasize the importance of the presence of a retrohyaloid hemorrhage at this point, which is an indication for surgery in a diabetic patient. To highlight the diabetic patient in whom a vitrectomy surgery is performed, the presence of rebleeding constrains us to the searchfor new vesels at the level of the sclerotomies, and it is often difficult and unsuccessful by ultrasound because their small size and flow make their detection impossible in many cases. The B-mode ultrasound shows an echogenic structure of triangular appearance, with its base toward the periphery of the eye.

4. Proliferative Diabetic Retinopathy

The presence of new vesels at the level of the papilla, vascular arcades, or optic disc [PDR], just like the presence of new vesels at the level of surgical sclerotomies performed during the vitrectomy can lead to the formation of vitreous hemorrhage. If there are vascular proliferations directed to the vitreous cavity, the ultrasound detects it as hyper reflective tufts that stick to the vitreous, slightly moving with the eye movement. Therefore, it is essential in these cases to observe the kinetic ultrasound to differentiate them from the vitreous bands adhered to the vitreous. In order to distinguish the presence of new vesels, we must use the Color-Doppler (Fig. **9**), which provides us information about the presence of hematic circulation in the observed vascular tufts [14]. In this section we include a highly destructive entity to the ocular globe, the anterior hyaloid fiber vascular proliferation, which can lead the eye to *phthisis bulbi*. Its appearance is not uncommon even after multiple vitrectomies. In ultrasound, we can observe the presence of a continuous, generally flat membrane, at the extreme periphery of the retina, many times just above the ciliary body with retinal tractions and adherence to the residual vitreous skirt. In these cases, an exploration alternative would be the use of scanning probes close to 20 MHz that would provide better detail of the structures located behind the iris.

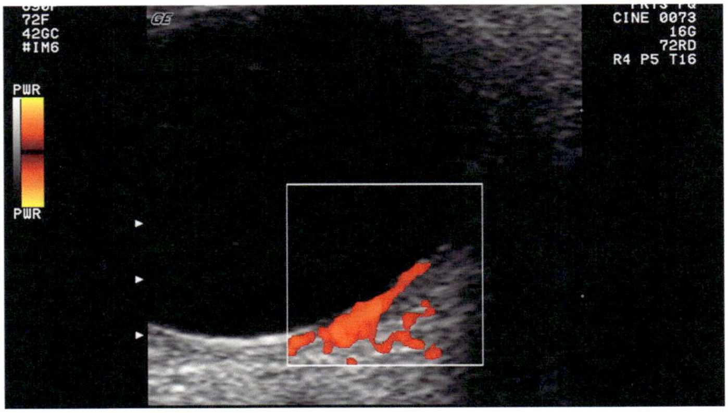

Figure 9: Proliferative diabetic retinopathy, we observe papillary new vessels.

5. Retinal Tractional Detachment

Through ultrasound, we can observe the presence of retinal lifting in very specific areas, being not much extensive and located near the posterior pole, but unlike the rhegmatogenous retinal detachment, it is much more stable and poorly movable in the kinetic ultrasound. If we closely observe the images, sometimes they have a peak shape, which in its most acute part closely adheres to the vitreous, by not being strange in the presence of vitreous fibres closely attached to the retina with scarce mobility (Fig. **10**). In more advanced stages, retinal detachment may be complete and take the form of a scarcely movable rigid funnel in the kinetic ultrasound.

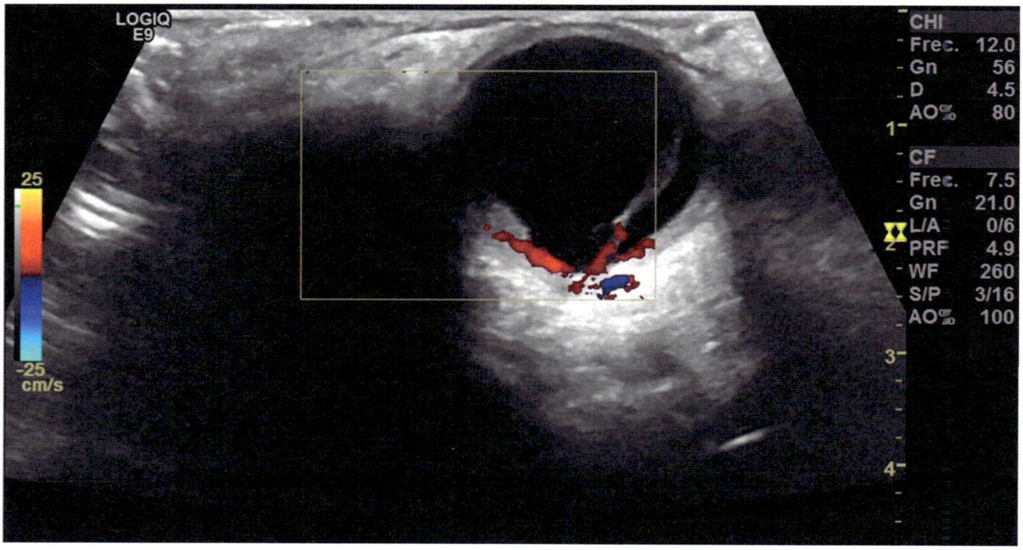

Figure 10: Tractional retinal detachment, induced by proliferative diabetic retinopathy. We can observe in color doppler the proliferative retinopathy with retinal traction.

6. Diabetic Macular Edema

Through ultrasound, we can observe the presence of thickening in the retinal wall at the macular level, if there is diabetic macular edema that translates to hyper reflectivity in that area. Projections are preferred upon the sclera [9 hours in the right eye and 3 hours in the left], and are non-axial in the study of the macular area because they avoid going through the cornea and the lens, giving a better picture of the macular area. The presence of tractions in the macular area can also be observed by ultrasound that can determine the source itself of the edema; and sometimes within the macular area, there may appear areas of hypo echogenicity corresponding to the presence of considerable size cysts inside the edema (Fig. **11**). Although the fluorescein angiography and the computed tomography [CT] are higher procedures to determine the presence of diabetic macular edema, these need to have a good transparent media and a proper pupil dilation, but in diabetic patients, the presence of vitreous opacities is not strange [for example: hemorrhages] [15, 16].

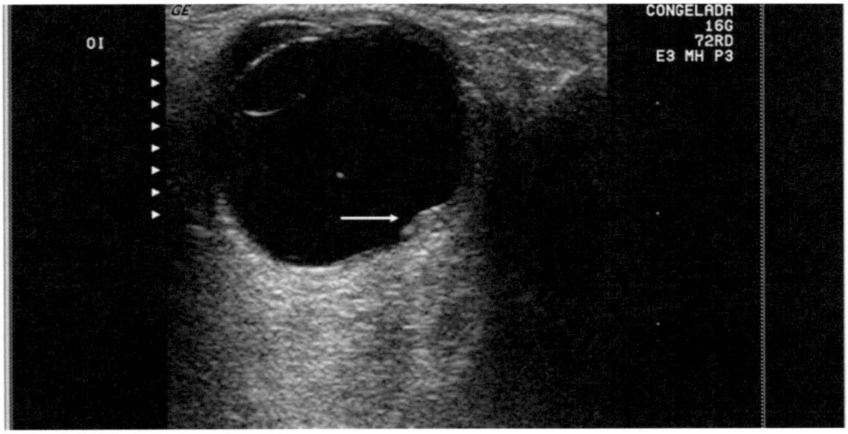

Figure 11: Diabetic macular edema, we can observe a thickening in macular area, which is a thickened diabetic macular upper to 1000μ.

CENTRAL RETINAL ARTERY OCCLUSION

The presence of a central retinal artery occlusion, or its branches, is easily diagnosed by its clinical features and the fundus examination, in which it shows the non-perfused area in the retina, and in many cases, the vascular occlusion area, usually by an embolus. The emboli can be: of platelet source [the most common source is an ulcerated carotid plaque in this case]; of cholesterol source, released from atheromatous plaque carotid; or of a secondary calcification source, usually from a valvular heart disease; less commonly, the emboli may occur from a tumors source or thrombocitary. The use of ocular echography, in these cases, is not usually necessary by the given permeability of the media to the display of the retina. However, in these cases, we found a decrease in the flow velocity of the central retinal artery using a Color-Doppler.

CENTRAL RETINAL VEIN OCCLUSION

It is the second leading cause of retinal vascular disease, after the diabetic retinopathy that includes central vein occlusions, of any of its branches, and the hemi-occlusions or the hemi-retinal occlusions. Central vein occlusions are the most frequent; the annual impact rate is 2-3 per 10,000 populations, being more frequent in men. It can occur in two clinical forms: an edematous form, or with normal blood perfusion, and the other being poor perfusion, or ischemic In the second case, the clinical presentation includes an important low visual acuity from the beginning. The first form of presentation described, the edematous or normal perfusion, may evolve to ischemia in a period of weeks or months; in this case, neovascularization can be developed at the level of the iris and trigger a secondary neovascular glaucoma. Unlike the previous case, it is not strange that the presence of vitreous hemorrhage appears with a central retinal vein occlusion; in this case, the ultrasound may be useful to us indeed. To explore vein occlusion by ultrasound, especially the form of central vein occlusion, we must perform a Color-Doppler ultrasound; a reduction of the diastolic peak velocity of the central retinal vein is observed in these patients (Fig. **12**). This determination is sign of a possible neovascularization manifestation in the iris, even if the velocity is less than 3.0 cm/sec [17].

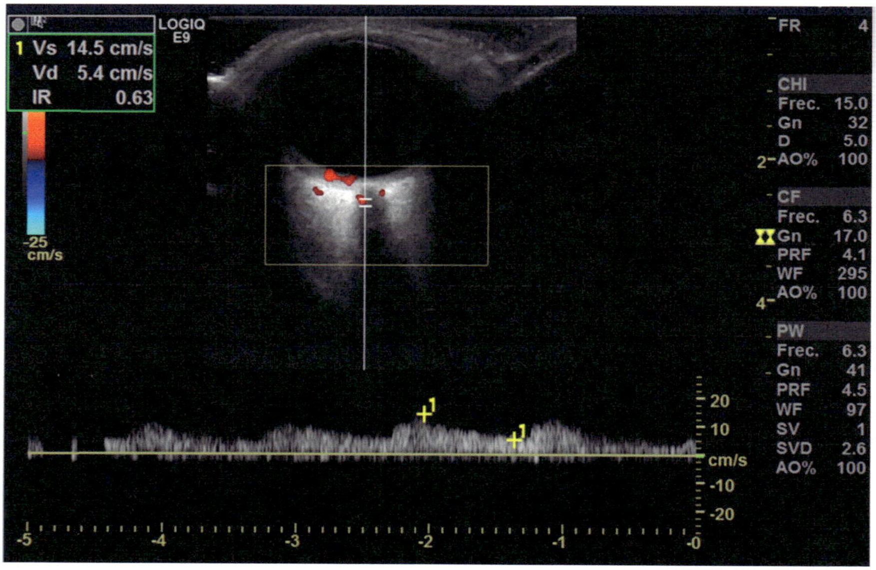

Figure 12: Color doppler in a case of central vein occlusion. Low diastolic peak.

VASCULAR INSUFFICIENCY [OPHTHALMIC AND CAROTID ARTERIES]

Carotid vascular insufficiency stems from a blood flow alteration in the level of the carotid common portion or in the level of the internal carotid or its first branch of the ophthalmic artery eye. Vascular insufficiency may have two origins: the release of emboli or the appearance of a low vascular output due to stenosis; in this case, the most common cause is atherosclerosis. Ocular vascular insufficiency gives the most important clinical sign to the apparition of an amaurosis fugax crisis of repetition; it appears in 60% of patients with carotid atheroma demonstrated by arteriography, and in the 80% of cases, it is demonstrated by carotid Color-Doppler ultrasound. Vision loss is severe, and it lasts 2 to 10 minutes approximately. The amaurosis fugax is the equivalent of the transient cerebral vascular insufficiency; and just like the latter mentioned, it carries a risk of subsequent ocular complications; thus the risk of vision loss, while low, is about 7%. The most common clinical conditions associated with ocular vascular insufficiency are: the chronic ischemic retinopathy, which is easily diagnosed with an ophthalmoscopy exam [dilated veins, nummular intraretinal hemorrhages, and microaneurysms], and the anterior segment ischemia syndrome [associated with: episcleral congestion, corneal edema, anterior chamber tyndall, unreactive pupil, rubeosis iridis, intraocular pressure changes sometimes high and sometimes too low]; this last picture is associated with angina pain in the eye. The ultrasound examination of the carotid vessels, and their branches, is currently the method of choice for its diagnosis [18-20]. If the occlusion is due to ophthalmic artery stenosis, we would be able to observe a decrease in its flow velocity values, by comparing it to the contralateral eye. It may also detect decreases in the flow of the central retinal artery and the posterior ciliary arteries. The study of the carotid arteries by ultrasound shows both early changes related with hypertrophy of the intima-media complex and the existence of plaques; its ultrasound characteristics and a percentage of stenosis. Stenosis greater than 50% will condition changes in the spectral morphology.

RETINAL DETACHMENT

The retina is a complex eye structure formed by several layers of cells responsible for collecting, processing and then transmitting the visual information from photoreceptors to the ganglion cells, the attachment where the optic nerve is formed. Thanks to its neurological nature, the retina is able to transform the light stimulus into an electrical phenomenon; this process is called visual phototransduction. In order to keep the neurosensory retina [NR] attached to the underlying layer, the retinal pigment epithelium [RPE], the proper functioning of a series of complementary mechanisms is necessary. The main mechanisms of adhesion are the pressure exerted by the vitreous on the retina.

Types of Retinal Detachment

- Retinal detachment [RD] is usually classified into three types according to the underlying etiopathogenic mechanism:
- Rhegmatogenous retinal detachment [RRD]
- Exudative retinal detachment [ERD]
- Tractional retinal detachment [TRD]

1. Rhegmatogenous Retinal Detachment [RRD]

The RRD is, by far, the most common of all of them. It is caused by a retinal tear resulting from a tangential vitreous traction on it. The liquefied vitreous and the aqueous humor filter themselves through the formed hole, and they detach progressively the RN from the RPE. The location of the retinal tear is usually anterior, at the back edge of the vitreous base. In high myopic eyes, the presentation of the retinal tear may be at a level more posterior due to the pathological adhesions of the posterior vitreous on the retina; by being characteristic of the retinal paravascular holes [21]. The RD by macular hole is characteristic of this group of patients.

2. Echography Usefulness in Rhegmatogenous Retinal Detachment

Despite the gradual appearance of new diagnostic tests in ophthalmology, the ocular ultrasound remains an important support tool in the management of RRD in skilled hands. It is useful in the following situations:

- Initial evaluation of the posterior segment of the eye.
- Monitoring and evolution of the postoperative retinal detachment.
- Evaluation of the scleral procedures.

Initial evaluation of the posterior segment of the eye: In certain situations, one suspects the coexistence of retinal pathology as a cause of low vision as well as media opacity caused by a cataract or any other reason (Fig. **13**). The most common reason is the mature cataract. Retinal pathology is ruled out all patients diagnosed with mature cataract who had a lower visual acuity than the hand movements. In this situation, the presence of an exudative macular degeneration or a chronic retinal detachment is common. In the latter case, ocular ultrasound helps establish the anatomic prognosis of the patient, by assessing: the location and extent of the DR, the retinal degree of stiffness, and the presence and location of the vitreoretinal proliferation [VRP]. Poor prognosis signs are: total retinal detachment, thickening of its thickness, the lack of mobility with the after movement technique and the presence of VRP grade D as shown by the classic funnel configuration of the retina (Fig. **14**). Patients who have suffered a severe blunt ocular trauma, with hyphema or resulting vitreous hemorrhage, require an ultrasound evaluation to assess the condition of the internal structures of the eye. By using ultrasound, we aim to assess: the ocular globe anatomic integrity, the condition of the lens-iris diaphragm, the intraocular lens location in pseudophakic patients, the presence of vitreous hemorrhage and the concomitant existence of choroid or retina.

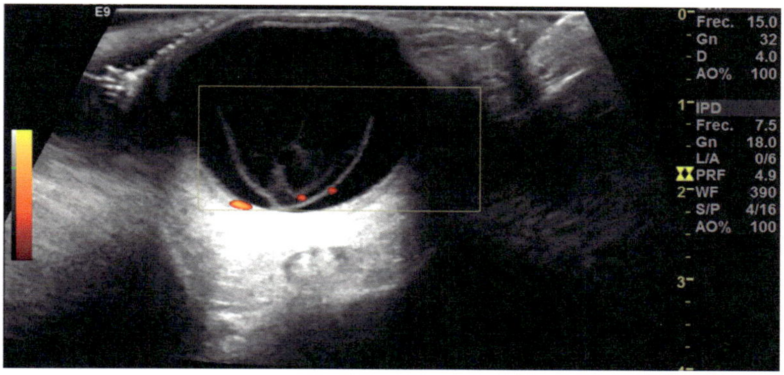

Figure 13: Retinal detachment, retina remain adhered in the papilla.

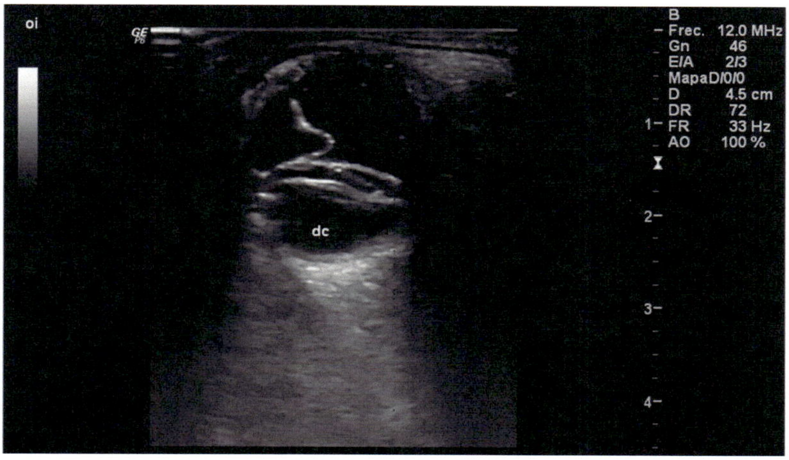

Figure 14: Proliferative vitreous retinopathy (PVR). In this case the retina is folded into a Greek Y, with a choroidal detachment (dc) inferiorly.

3. Retinal Detachment Post-Operative Monitoring

Some RD operated patients develop cataracts at an early stage in the first month after surgery. Mainly, it is in those patients on whom a pars plana vitrectomy is performed. Another risk factor for its development is the iatrogenic contact of the lens with the stems of the surgical instruments not facilitating the patient in correct positioning, in the post-operative period. Secondary cataract sometimes can prevent the proper fundoscopic monitoring of the retina. It is in these cases in which an ultrasound follow-up is required to objectify, the right anatomical condition, until a cataract surgery is performed. As long as there remains gas in the posterior segment, ultrasound is recommended in a sitting position in order to optimize the quality of the images obtained.

4. Evaluation of Scleral Procedures

Despite of the undergone progress of the posterior vitrectomy in recent years, the scleral buckle remains, in some cases, the technique of choice for the treatment of RD. By using ultrasound, we can observe the scleral procedures location, and the presence of inflammation signs characterized by thickening, vascularity rising in Color-Doppler study and the presence of collections. It is also possible to evaluate the subsequent migration of the episcleral bands.

EXUDATIVE RETINAL DETACHMENT [ERD]

The ERD is caused by an accumulation of fluid between the NR and the RPE in the absence of retinal hole. The ERD can be caused by various kinds of diseases. The most common are:

- Systemic metabolic diseases.
- Tumors and retinal vascular diseases.
- Posterior uveitis. Posterior scleritis.
- Tumors and choroidal metastases.
- Tumors and congenital anomalies of the optic nerve.

Various metabolic disorders can cause disruption of the inner blood-retinal barrier [inner BRB] [retinal circulation] or the external blood-retinal barrier [EBRB] [constituted by the RPE], resulting in fluid manifestation between the NR and the

RPE. The most common cause is diabetes, by causing diffuse macular edema. Other causes include severe hypertension, eclampsia and renal insufficiency. Certain tumors and retinal vascular diseases may cause ERD by zonal functional incompetence of the retinal blood vessels and subsequent fluid accumulation. It is the case of Coats disease that typically causes a unilateral ERD in childhood. Another cause is the retinal capillary hemangioma that causes an ERD with the presence of perilesional lipid exudation. The infectious or inflammatory chorioretinitis may cause an alteration of the inner BRB and EBRB generating an ERD due to the released inflammatory mediators. The presence of multiple ERD in the posterior pole is very characteristic of the Harada disease and the sympathetic ophthalmia. It is worth noting that posterior scleritis by secondarily chorio-retinal inflammation can cause unilateral or bilateral ERD. In this case, ocular echography is useful to objectify both a scleral thickening increase and a vascular increase on Color-Doppler, which in addition with moderate to severe eye pain, is diagnostic of this disease. Some tumors such as choroidal hemangioma, melanoma, metastases and exceptionally the nevus, can cause a peritumoral retinal detachment more or less extensively (Fig. **15**). The main use of ultrasound, in this section, has helped establish the differential diagnosis between a melanoma and an exudative nevus, discarding the characteristic echographic signs of melanoma, such as choroidal excavation, orbital shadow and vascularization of the tumor. Some tumors and congenital anomalies of the optic nerve generate ERD. Thus, the papillary capillary hemangioma, especially those located at a temporal level, cause a macular ERD with high frequency. Doppler ultrasound reveals the tumor vascular nature. Among the congenital anomalies of the optic nerve that may cause an ERD at a macular level, the optic pit and coloboma stand out. Finally, entities of idiopathic nature, such as central serous chorioretinopathy or the uveal effusion syndrome, can generate an ERD more or less extensively.

TRACTIONAL RETINAL DETACHMENT [TRD]

The third type of retinal detachment is called tractional [TRD]. It occurs when the retina undergoes a centripetal force greater than that exerted in all the adhesion mechanisms to the underlying RPE. This type of RD usually occurs in the ischemic retinopathies, in which fibrovascular proliferations [FVP] are generated and during their evolution, suffer shrinkage phenomena, by being at this stage when they produce the greatest traction on the retina (Fig. **18**). Again, diabetes is the most common cause. Other causes include the retinal vasculitis and the sickle-cell anemia.

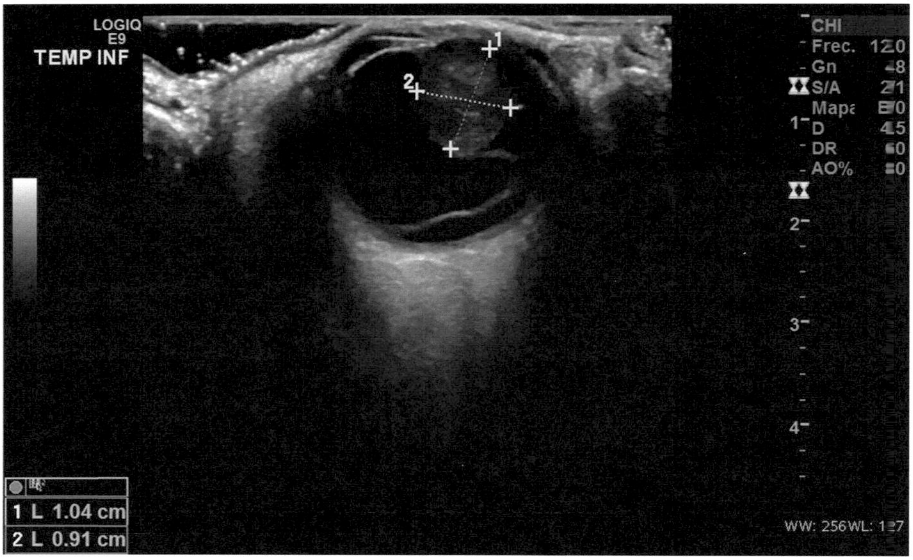

Figure 15: Exudative retinal detachment induced by melanoma.

1. Echography Usefulness in the Tractional Retinal Detachment [TRD]

The main indication for ocular ultrasound, in the study of the patient in whom a TRD has been suspected, is the inability to properly visualize the posterior segment because of media opacity. The most common reason is the presence of hemovitreous. After the diagnosis is confirmed, ocular ultrasound helps establish the patient's visual prognosis by evaluating whether TRD affects the macula, or is peripheral, its size and the concomitant presence of an RRD.

MACULAR PATHOLOGY

The macular area study is usually performed under direct vision, either by ophthalmoscopy, posterior biomicroscopy using lenses of +90 diopters, fundography, or by optical tomography [OT]. But if the media are opaque and make the visualization of the posterior pole difficult, ultrasound can help: in this case, we have to use probes of 10 MHz or 20 MHz. With a relatively low gain, we are able to study the eye wall; and with a high gain, we can study the vitreo-retinal interface [22].

1. Macular Hole

The 10 MHz ultrasound allows us to properly observe macular holes of stages III and IV, while with probes of 20 MHz, we can refine the diagnosis to a greater extent [23]. The ring-shaped serous detachment of the retinal epithelium is reflected by a highly echogenic macular protrusion, with a small central depression that corresponds to the retinal defect. The vitreo-retinal interface is difficult to observe by ultrasound despite the increase in gain and noise, making it difficult to observe the existence of posterior vitreous detachment as close to the retina. The high retinal operculum is a small hyper-echogenic nodule around the hole. Stage II holes are much more difficult to observe, and stage I holes are impossible to detect using ultrasound. In the presence of macular hole in one eye, it is essential to study the contralateral eye in order to detect the presence of posterior vitreous detachment, because there is a high risk of a macular hole formation in the eye,; in its absence, such exploration can be done by using ultrasound and high gain.

2. Epimacular Membranes

It is very hard to assess the presence of epiretinal membranes by using ultrasound, especially at 10 MHz, only with frequencies near to 20 MHz an increase of reflectivity in the macular area can be observed.

3. Retinal-Traction Syndromes

By using probes of 10 MHz and 20 MHz, a macular area thickening associated with a highly reflective and thickened hyaloid attached to the macular area can be observed.

4. Serous Detachment of the Retinal Pigment Epithelium

In serous detachment or the retinal pigment epithelium we can see a small membrane with respect to the ocular wall, at the macular area. In case of doubt, the successive performance of scans can help to differentiate the injuries described above.

CHOROIDAL PATHOLOGY

1. Choroidal Thickening

According to ultrasound scan, the total ocular wall thickness [retina, choroid and sclera] varies from 1 mm to 2.5 mm in the myopia, in the farsighted; and approximately, 1.5 mm in the emmetrope. The choroidal thickness varies between 0.5 and 1 mm at the posterior pole. Sometimes we find a choroidal thickness growth that we always must distinguish a tumor cause [choroidal melanoma, lymphoma, or metastasis].

The entities, which may provide choroidal diffuse thickening are:

- Ocular hypotony
- Swellings [Posterior uveitis or choroiditis]
- Lymphoid hyperplasia
- Endophthalmitis
- Post traumatic ocular venous return occlusion [orbital tumor, carotid-cavernous fistula]; in the course of an ocular trauma, a located or diffuse choroidal thickening may occur, which, being more than 2 mm, may be taken as a progression sign for ocular atrophy [phthisis bulbi]

The entities which may provide located choroidal thickening are:

- Vitreo-retinal traction
- Located suprachoroidal small hemorrhages [choroidal hematoma]
- Presence of an embedded foreign body in the ocular wall
- Berlin's edema [post contusive macular edema]
- Choroidal dehiscence

2. Choroidal Thinning

The choroidal and ocular wall thinning may show up in a congenital way, but its association with the high axial myopia is more common. In this latter entity, we can observe the formation of posterior staphyloma, which are visible in ultrasound in the form of posterior bulging in the ocular wall, with choroidal and retinal thinning; in these cases, it is possible to observe, at the vitreous level, its full or partial detachment. In the latter case, we observe vitreous tracts attached to the posterior ocular wall.

3. Serous Choroidal Detachment

The formation of a serous choroidal detachment can show up in different entities:

- After any eye surgery which involves the ocular globe opening, with the resulting intra-ocular hypotension. Above all, it may occur in case of cataract surgery, being more frequently in those surgeries with intraoperative complications, or if the technique performed is extra capsular, or well during or after glaucoma surgery [trabeculectomy] where postoperative hypotension is frequent.

- During the course of an orbital or intraocular swelling [*e.g.* uveitis]
- After an eye injury involving or not the ocular globe
- Spontaneously

On examination by ultrasound, we can observe the presence of a regular and convex bulging in the direction of the eye socket (Fig. **16**). This regularity and convexity combined with a low mobility of an over raised area is what highlights the difference between a serous detachment from a retinal detachment (Fig. **17**). Usually, the location is set from the release of the vorticose veins, in its most posterior portion, to the scleral spur, in its most anterior portion. We can also observe that the posterior ocular wall of the bulging area is thinner than the not lifted ocular wall; the wall thickness difference at the detachment starting area is called "sep-sign". The detachment content is completely anechogenic; although, sometimes, undefined echoes are observed in its interior. The most important differential diagnosis is the retinal detachment as mentioned above, but the signs described above, as well the fact that the retinal detachment occurs with a much more irregular wall, sometimes thickened if it is old, and which adheres to the papilla [in the choroidal detachment rarely goes beyond the vorticose veins], allow its differentiation (Fig. **18**).

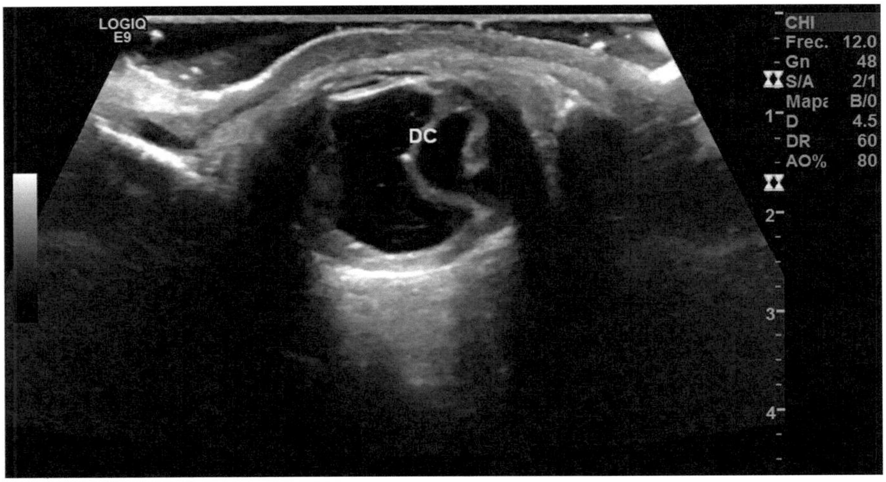

Figure 16: Choroidal detachment (DC), secondary to intraocular hypotension after vitrectomy

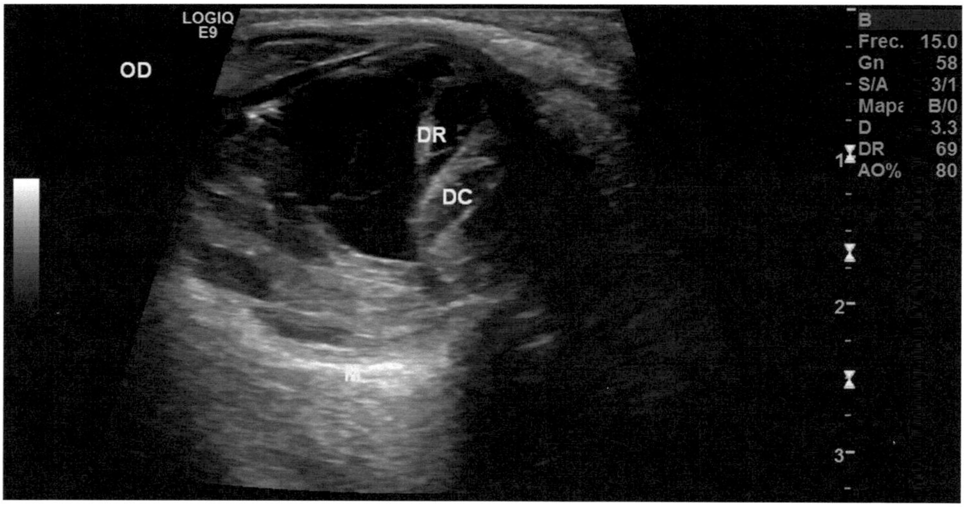

Figure 17: Retinal detachment (DR), and choroidal detachment (DC).

4. Suprachoroidal Hemorrhage

The presence of a suprachoroidal origin hemorrhage is the result of the long ciliary vessels rupture that passes just beneath the sclera and above the choroid; besides, these vessels are closely linked to the sclera by connective junctions that impede its elongation or resizing. The hemorrhage formation in this space is usually caused by a surgical procedure involving ocular globe opening, as in the case of cataract surgery. By using ultrasound, one is able to see a choroidal bulging in the hemorrhage area, with a heterogeneous echogenic aspect, which is denser and compact in the first days after the appearance of the hemorrhage (Fig. **18**); and as days pass by, it begins to liquefy forming cavities less reflective to ultrasound inside the hemorrhage area (Fig. **19**). It is important to rule out the presence of associated retinal detachment with ultrasound, and if it has formed two prominent bags that come in contact with each other at the level of the vitreous cavity, the choroidal hemorrhage kiss (Fig. **20**) is an important finding, which may indicate an emergency surgery to prevent the unions appearance between both retinas that unlikely would be split up during surgery [24, 25]. Currently, the suprachoroidal hemorrhage treatment to follow is vitreous surgery. If this hemorrhage is important and is not spontaneously reabsorbed, the performed technique will include the performing of sclerotomy drainage, which will require the presence of hemorrhage liquefaction. Therefore, it is necessary to perform ultrasound scans in the course of the days after the hemorrhage in order to observe the appearance of such liquefaction areas previously described, which usually appear between the seventh and fourteenth day after the hemorrhage.

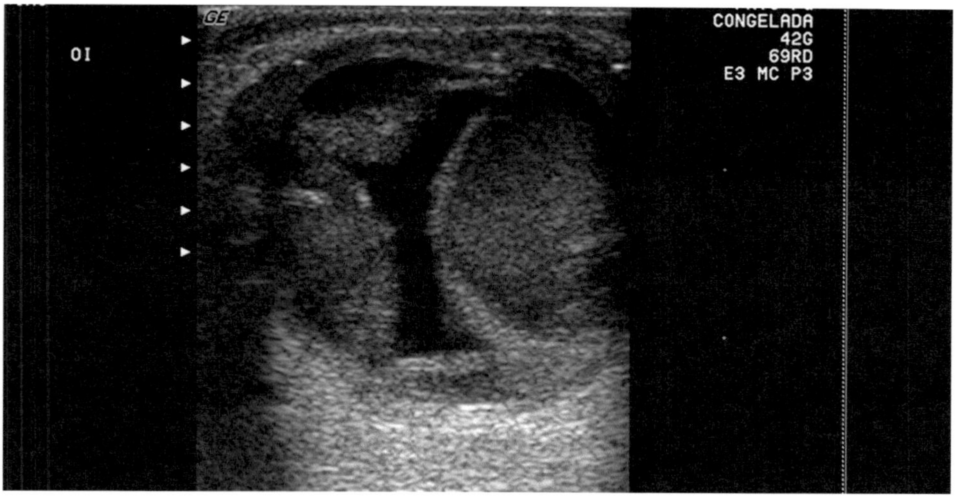

Figure 18: Supra choroidal hemorrhage.

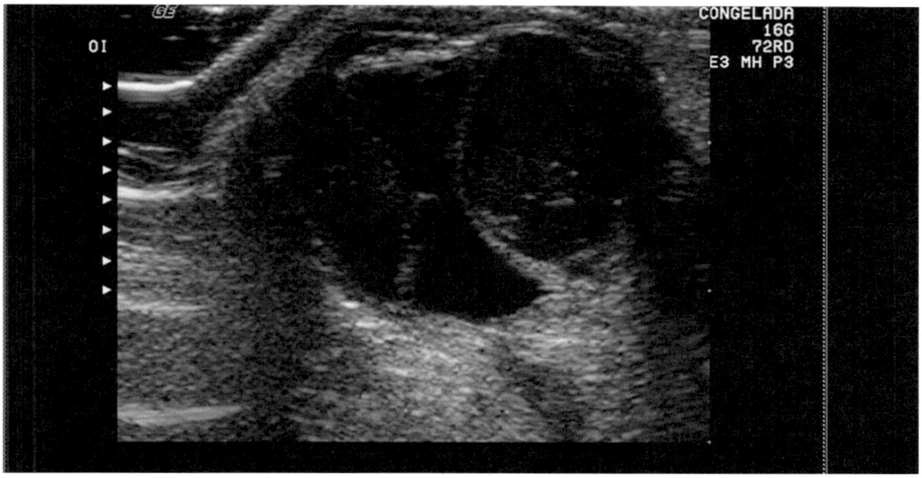

Figure 19: The same case of Fig. **18**, a case of supra choroidal hemorrhage in reabsorption.

SCLERAL PATHOLOGY

1. Inflammatory Disturbances

The most frequent pathological entity affecting the sclera is its inflammation; its classification would be:

- Episcleritis: inflammation of the superficial layers of the sclera; it commonly affects the anterior portion located beneath the conjunctiva, without affecting the posterior portion of the ocular globe.

- Nodular, nodular and focal episcleral involvement

- Diffuse, episcleral diffuse involvement scleritis, involvement of the entire scleral thickness, can be:

    - Anterior scleritis: it affects the anterior portion of the ocular globe.

    - Posterior scleritis: it affects the posterior portion of the ocular globe.

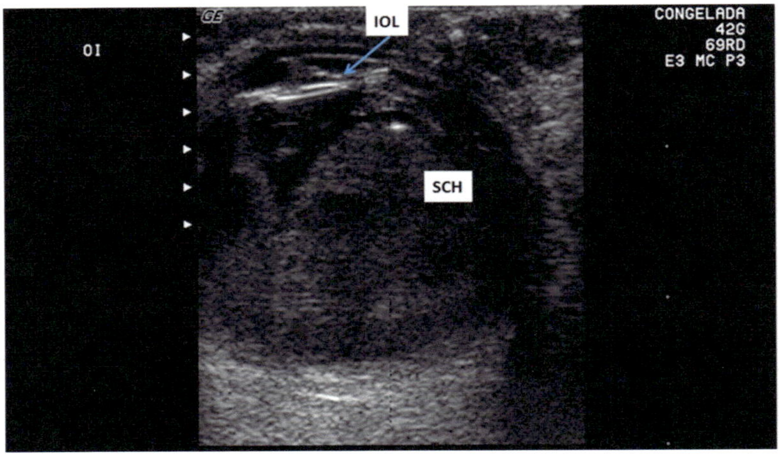

Figure 20: Kiss sign in a double supra choroidal hemorrhage (SCH), in a patient operated of cataract surgery with an intraocular lens (IOL).

Additionally, a nodular and a diffuse form of scleritis may appear, like the episcleritis, associated with any of the two previous forms. The episcleritis and scleritis above are easily diagnosed by anterior segment biomicroscopy, but not the following involvement of the scleritis can be associated with an earlier form. Thus, before any form of scleritis with or without previous involvement, an ultrasound scan of the posterior segment is not advisable. In the ultrasound, we observe a thickening of the posterior ocular wall, especially due to a growth in the sclera thickness that is manifested in the form of a heterogeneous hyperechogenicity of the sclera; these findings also include a choroidal thickening and an edema, or Tenon's capsule swelling, that we observe as a thin hypoechoic layer at the back of the sclera with some bond angles to the ocular wall at the entrance level of the optic nerve to the eye, being very sharp in a T shape form. The differential diagnosis includes ocular lymphoma, but in this the thickening is much more important, and the Tenon bond angles are softer and less acute. In case of located or nodular involvement of posterior scleritis, the differential diagnosis includes intraocular tumors, but the use of ultrasound, in these cases, is less useful; and therefore requires other diagnostic imaging.

2. Scleral Thinning

The scleral and ocular wall thinning is usually associated with high axial myopia. In this latter entity, we can observe the formation of posterior staphyloma (Figs. **21**, **22**), which are visible in ultrasound in the form of posterior bulging in the ocular wall, with choroidal and retinal thinning; the antero-posterior axis is increased, and the posterior bulging in the ocular wall is not often uniform across the posterior wall, but rather it forms a kind of tunnel at a superior level many times.

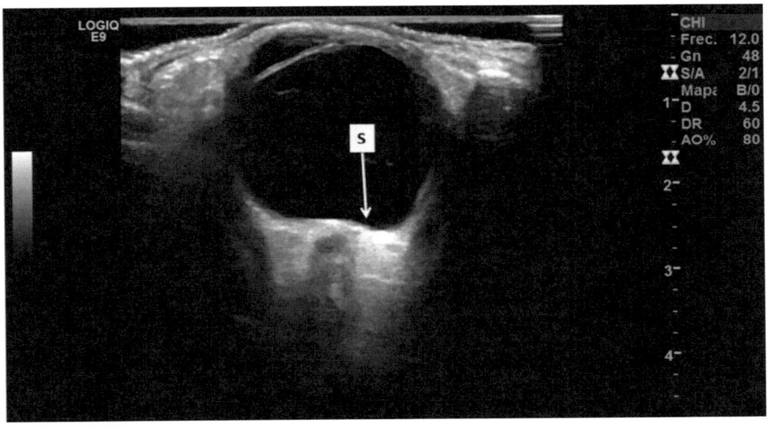

Figure 21: Myopic staphiloma (S).

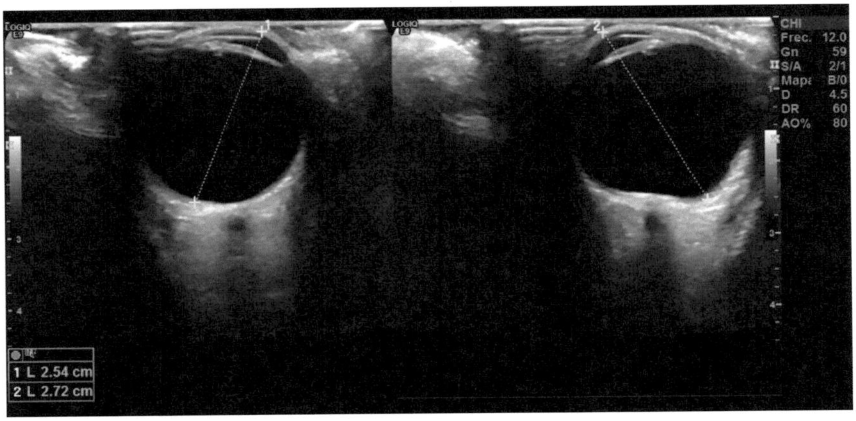

Figure 22: Axial myopia in both eyes [eye normal length = 2.2], with staphiloma in right eye.

PAPILLARY PATHOLOGY

By using ultrasound, the entrance of the optic nerve to the ocular wall can be seen as a biconvex protrusion with a small central depression [papillary excavation]; these observations are more evident with the 20 MHz probe. On the contrary, in order to observe the ocular globe posterior portion, it is necessary to use a 10 MHz probe, which allows us to study the retrobulbar portion located at the back of the cribriform plate; and by ultrasound, the optic nerve ultrasound appears as an elongated hypoechoic structure and the meninges appear that cover it up as a hypo-echogenic form. The optic nerve situation is nasal related to the ocular globe [26].

1. Papilledema

It may be observed that the formed protrusion by the optic nerve inside the vitreous cavity is increased with a decreased echostructure. In case of fluid accumulation in the subarachnoid space [by an intracerebral pressure increase for example], a separation at the level of the hyper-echogenic layers that surrounds the optic nerve is observed.

2. Optic Nerve Tumors

Some tumors, like the retinoblastoma or the ocular melanoma, can spread themselves into the optic nerve [these tumors are described in their corresponding chapters], and equally the meningiomas and gliomas of the optic nerve can be observed in the retrobulbar area of the same [its description is not described in this book, because it stands at the orbital region]. The melanocytoma is a special case; a tumor located in the papilla can be seen as a hyper-echogenic injury, located on small papilla bulging into the vitreous cavity with 20 MHz probe being a more evident mass lesion [27].

3. Drusen

Drusen, at papillary level of the optic nerve, can be observed as hyper-echogenic nodules that form a posterior acoustic shadow cone to them, especially if they are calcified (Fig. **23**).

4. Papillary Excavation Study

There is a high correlation degree between an OCT and an ultrasound, mainly at 20 MHz in the papillary morphological study. The physiological papillary excavation is clearly visible by ultrasound in the form of a small central depression. The rise of this depression can be seen on ultrasound as a central depression rise that is able to eliminate the intraocular profusion of the optic nerve in advanced cases, by being able to form an authentic pot shape. Also, if there is atrophy of the optic nerve, one can observe the presence of a hypoechoic area lower than 3 mm, at the papillary level of the optic nerve, corresponding to an absence of fiber [normally, the fiber thickness in the ultrasound is between 3 mm and 3.6 mm]. The Color-Doppler ultrasound study allows to note the vascularization absence around the papilla in case of optic nerve atrophy [28, 29].

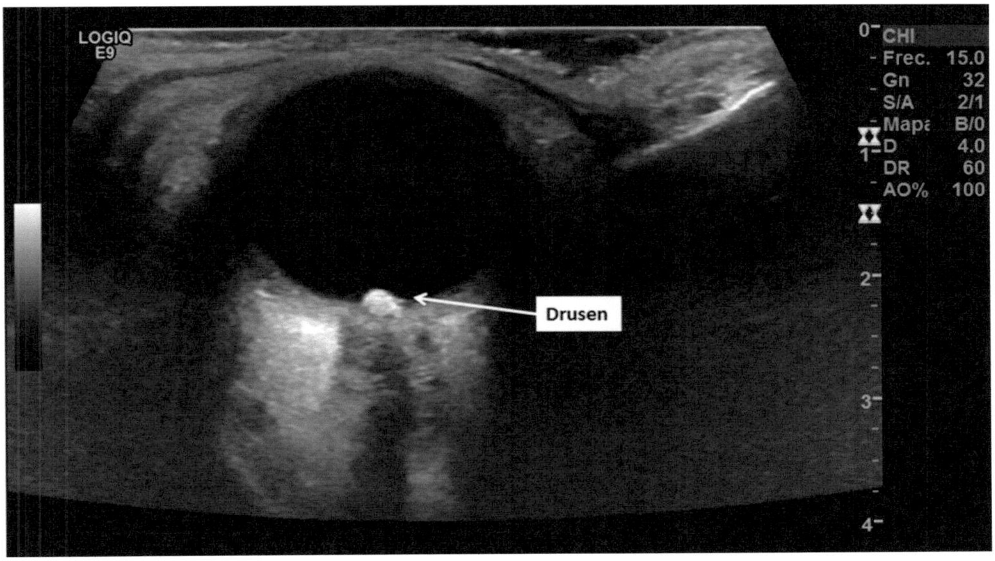

Figure 23: Papillary drusen.

CONCLUDING REMARKS

The 15 to 20 MHz ultrasounds are an important technique of posterior segment examination. A multiple of ocular pathologies of vitreous, retina, choroid and sclera are diagnosed with echography. In cases of cataract or other media opacities, the echography helps to correct diagnosis of ocular pathologies as retinal detachment, diabetic retinopathy, vasculopathies as venous occlusion, and a great number of choroid and sclera diseases. Furthermore, the ultrasound is important in the diagnosis of optic nerve disorders.

ACKNOWLEDGEMENTS

Declared None.

CONFLICT OF INTEREST

The authors confirm that this chapter contents have no conflict of interest.

REFERENCES

[1] Kubal WS. The pathological globe: clinical and imaging analysis. Semin Ultrasound CT MR. 1997; 18 (6): 423-36.

[2] Fielding JA. Ocular ultrasound.Clin Radiol. 1996; 51(8): 533-44.

[3] Testut L, Latarjet A. Anatomía Humana. Capítulo IV Sentido de la vista. Editorial SALVAT SA Barcelona 1980. Pag 555-729.

[4] Bair RL, Wells RG, Massaro BM, *et al*. Imaging in orbital trauma. Semin Ophthalmol. 1994; 9(3): 185-92.

[5] Fielding JA. Imaging the eye with ultrasound.Br J Hosp Med. 1992 Jun 3-16; 47(11): 805-15.

[6] Lieb WE. Color-Doppler imaging of the eye and orbit. Radiol Clin North Am. 1998; 36(6): 1059-71.

[7] MacKinnon JR, McKillop G, O'Brien C, *et al*. Color-Doppler imaging of the ocular circulation in diabetic retinopathy. Acta Ophthalmol Scand. 2000; 78(4): 386-9.

[8] Bedi DG, Gombos DS, Ng CS, *et al*. Echography of the eye. AJR Am J Roentgenol. 2006; 187(4): 1061-72.

[9] Luna JD, Artal MN, Reviglio VE, *et al*. Vitreoretinal alterations following laser in situ keratomileusis: clinical and experimental studies. Graefes Arch Clin Exp Ophthalmol. 2001; 239: 416-23.

[10] Lavric A, Urbancic M. Floating vitreous cyst: two clinical cases. Case Rep Ophthalmol. 2013 8; 4(3): 243-7.

[11] Gavrilov JC, Gaujoux T, Sellam M, *et al*. Occurrence of posterior vitreous detachment after femtosecond laser in situ keratomileusis: Ultrasound evaluation. J Cataract Refract Surg. 2011; 37(7): 1300-4.

[12] Zvornicanin J, Jusufovic V, Cabric E, Musanovic Z, Zvornicanin E, Popovic-Beganovic A. Significance of echography in evaluation of vitreo-retinal pathologies. Med Arh. 2012; 66(5): 318-20.

[13] Chu TG, Lopez PF, Cano MR, Freeman WR, *et al*. Posterior vitreoschisis. An echographic finding in proliferative diabetic retinopathy. Ophthalmology. 1996; 103(2): 315-22.

[14] Karami M, Janghorbani M, Dehghani A, *et al*. Orbital Doppler evaluation of blood flow velocities in patients with diabetic retinopathy. Rev Diabet Stud. 2012; 9(2-3): 104-11.

[15] Arai T, Numata K, Tanaka K, *et al*. Ocular arterial flow hemodynamics in patients with diabetes mellitus. J Ultrasound Med. 1998; 17: 675—81.

[16] Langham ME, Grebe R, Hopkins S, *et al*. Choroidal blood flow in diabetic retinopathy. Exp Eye Res. 1991; 52: 167-73.

[17] Schicke SH, Duncker GI. Retinal Color-Doppler scanning of arteria centralis retinae by retinal diseases and healthy people. Klin Monbl Augenheilkd. 2007; 224(10): 775-9.

[18] Turek G, Kochanowicz J, Rutkowski R, *et al* Accuracy of transcranial colour-coded echography in the diagnosis of anterior cerebral artery vasospasm. Neurol Neurochir Pol. 2012; 46(3): 233-8.

[19] Barnes RW, Ross EA, Strandness DE Jr. Differntiation of primary from secondary varicose veins by Doppler ultrasound and strain gauge plethysmography. Surg Gynecol Obstet. 1975; 141(2): 207-11.

[20] Thiele BL, Young JV, Chikos PM, *et al*. Correlation of arteriographic findings and symptoms in cerebrovascular disease. Neurology. 1980; 30(10): 1041-6.

[21] Shimada N, Ohno-Matsui K, Nishimuta A, *et al*. Detection of lamellar holes and other paravascular by optical coherent tomography Abnormalities in eyes with high myopia. Ophthalmology 2008 Apr; 115 (4): 708-717.

[22] Zvornicanin J, Jusufovic V, Cabric E, *et al*. Significance of echography in evaluation of vitreo-retinal pathologies. Med Arh. 2012; 66(5): 318-20.

[23] Bottós JM, Torres VL, Kanecadan LA, *et al*. Macular hole: 10 and 20-MHz ultrasound and spectral-domain optical coherence tomography. Arq Bras Oftalmol. 2012; 75(6): 415-9.

[24] Feretis E, Mourtzoukos S, Mangouritsas G, *et al.* Secondary management and outcome of massive suprachoroidal hemorrhage. Eur J Ophthalmol. 2006; 16(6): 835-40.
[25] Sharma YR, Gaur A, Azad RV. Suprachoroidal hemorrhage. Secondary management. Indian J Ophthalmol. 2001; 49(3): 191-2.
[26] Lorente-Ramos RM, Armán JA, Muñoz-Hernández A, *et al.* Use of the eye made easy: a comprehensive how-to review with ophthalmoscopic correlation. Radiographics. 2012; 32(5): 175-200.
[27] Forte R, Cennamo G, Breve MA. Three-dimensional ultrasound of ophthalmic pathologies. Ophthalmologica. 2009; 223(3): 183-7.
[28] Braband K, Kerty E, Jakobsen JA. Contrast enhanced ultrasound Doppler examination of the retrobulbar arteries. Acta Radiol 2001; 42: 135.
[29] Harris A, Kagemann L, Cioffi G. Assessment of human ocular hemodynamics. Surv Ophthalmol 1998; 42: 509.

Chapter 5: Ocular Tumors

CHAPTER 5

Ocular Tumors

Marc Baget-Bernaldiz[1,*], Nuria Soler[1] and Manuel Montero-Jaime[2,*]

[1]Department of Ophthalmology, [2]Department of Radiology, University Hospital Sant Joan, Rovira & Virgili University, Pere Virgili Health Research Institute, IISPV, Reus, Spain

Abstract: The posterior segment tumors are the most important indication for ultrasound examination. Echography is essential in choroid melanoma diagnosis; there are a lot of signs in echography which permit us to make a differential diagnosis with the other most frequent intraocular tumor, metastases which appeared with similar echographic signs in ultrasound examination. In the present chapter we also explain the characteristics of other tumors, as retinoblastoma or choroid hemangioms.

Keywords: Choroid melanoma, retinoblastoma, choroid hemangioma, retina hemangioma, osteoma, metastases, astrocytic hamartoma.

INTRODUCTION

Frequently, the intraocular tumors are settled in the posterior pole of the eye. According to their nature there are several types of intraocular tumors: vascular tumors [choroidal hemangioma], glial type tumors [retinal astrocytic hamartoma], melanin type tumors [melanoma and choroidal nevus], mixed type tumors [combined hamartoma of the retina and the retinal pigment epithelium], or composed by foreign cells [choroidal metastases, primary ocular lymphoma]. Luckily for the ophthalmologist, most posterior pole tumors are presented under a characteristic that can be diagnosed quite easily. However, sometimes we have serious doubts about the tumor nature, and we have to use additional tests to try to establish the conclusive diagnosis. Some of these supplementary diagnostic tests are: intravenous fluoresce in angiography [IVFA], indocyanine green angiography [ICG], optical coherence tomography [OCT], ocular echography, computerized tomography [CT], magnetic resonance imaging [MRI], and finally ocular biopsy. Despite all these new diagnostic techniques available today, the ocular ultrasound assessment remains essential in the study of the tumors of the posterior pole.

***Corresponding author Marc Baget-Bernaldiz:** Hospital Universitario Sant Joan, Avda. Doctor Josep Laporte 1 Reus, Spain; E-mail: mbaget@grupsagessa.com
Pedro Romero Aroca: Hospital Universitario Sant Joan, Avda. Doctor Josep Laporte 1 Reus, Spain; E-mail: pormero@grupsagessa.com

Pedro Romero-Aroca and Manuel Montero-Jaime (Eds.)

TUMORS IN ECHOGRAPHY: B-MODE ECHOGRAPHY, A-MODE, AND COLOR-DOPPLER ULTRASOUND

The information obtained from each of them is intended to be complementary. Therefore the B-mode ultrasound studies the tumor nature, the tumor size, and the anatomical relationships with the ocular surrounding structures and the presence or absence of exudative retinal detachment. By using A-mode ultrasound, we obtain the internal reflectivity of the tumor, thus inferring its nature. Finally, by using the Color-Doppler ultrasound, it shows the amount of its vascularization.

CHOROID

1. Choroidal Hemangioma

Choroidal hemangioma is a benign tumor of vascular nature involving the middle layer [choroid] of the eye. This tumor can be of two forms: circumscribed [CCH] and diffuse. This latter, which is referred as the extent of the tumor greater than the fifty percent of the choroidal surface, almost exclusively affects patients with Sturge Weber syndrome [1]. CCH is much more common and is presented as an orange color lesion slightly hypochromic regarding the rest of the choroid. The differential diagnosis must be made with amelanotic choroidal melanoma and choroidal metastases [2]. The CCH is usually diagnosed between the third and fifth life decades [3]. It is usually asymptomatic, but when it is accompanied by serous exudation affecting the macula, metamorphopsia, loss of vision and hypermetropic shift has been described. The IVFA and ocular ultrasound are the two most useful medical tests in CCH. The IVFA allows outline the tumor contours from the retinal fundus. In A-mode ocular echography, we see a large initial echo corresponding to the anterior surface of the tumor, followed by several echoes with internal reflectivity between 50% and 100%, characteristic of the highly vascular tumors. In the B-mode ocular echography we cans see a highly acoustic lesion without posterior shadowing. Using Color-Doppler ultrasound the vascular nature of the tumor can be seen.

2. Choroidal Nevus

The choroidal nevus is the most common benign tumor of the posterior segment of the eye, which occurs up to 6.5% of the population [5]. Usually the diagnosis is not so difficult, but it always must be distinguish from choroidal melanoma [6, 7]. The importance of the absence of acoustic signal is a feature that has not been particularly emphasized for early detection of choroidal melanoma [8, 9]. However, according to Carol *et al.,* [10], approximately the 25% of all choroidal nevi with no acoustic signal at ultrasound assessment, could developed a choroidal melanoma. When a doubt therefore remains on diagnosis of choroidal nevus a fluorescein angiography [FA] and ultrasonographic study should be worked out. If the FA shows a hypofluorescence lesion with no vascularization signs, it is clear that we are facing a choroidal nevus. Using B-mode ultrasound we observe a slightly raised lesion with posterior shadowing. Color-Doppler does not observe tumor vascularization.

3. Choroidal Melanoma

Choroidal melanoma is the most common primary intraocular tumor in adults. It is usually diagnosed in the sixth decade of life by coincidence on routine examination. It could also be suspected by one of these symptoms: vision loss, floaters, metamorphopsia and even neovascular glaucoma in advanced cases. Usually presents as a dome shaped single lesion, dark brown or black colored, between the equator and the posterior pole. If they grow causing the Bruch's membrane to break, acquires the typical shape of mushroom or button down shirt. The visual and vital prognosis depends on tumor size [11, 12]. The FA and ocular ultrasound again becomes the two most useful medical tests to support the diagnosis. Dome tumors show a mottled fluorescence staining and progressive extravasation at early times. In the mushroom-shaped melanomas, we can see a dual circulation pattern, consisting of the presence of retinal and tumor vascularization. An ultrasound configuration of "shirt button" is almost pathognomonic for choroidal melanoma (Figs. **1**, **2**). The presence of acoustic shadowing and scleral excavation are characteristic signs of choroidal melanoma [13, 14]. The ultrasound Color-Doppler mode, demonstrates clearly a significant tumoral vascularity (Fig. **3**).

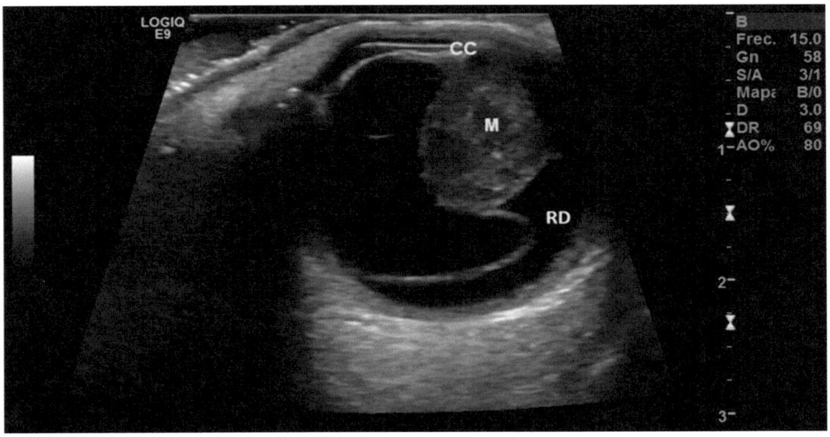

Figure 1: Choroidal melanoma (M), with secondary retinal detachment (RD), and cilliar body invasion (CC).

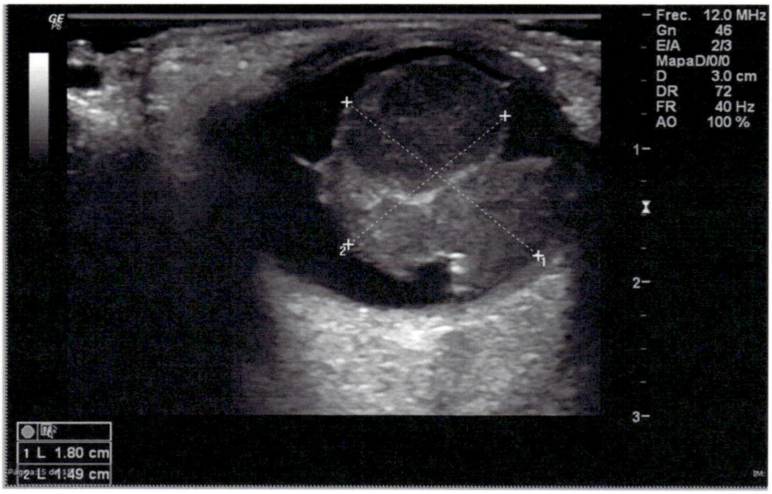

Figure 2: Mushroom choroidal melanoma

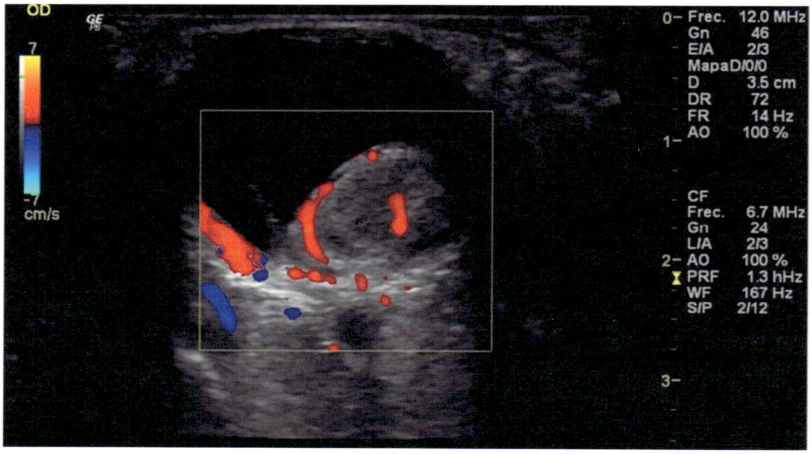

Figure 3: Color doppler of a choroidal melanoma, we observe the intra-tumor circulation.

4. Choroidal Osteoma

Choroidal osteoma is a benign tumor of unusual presentation, which consists in matured bone replacing choroidal tissue. It mainly affects middle-aged women and is located at juxtapapillary area [15]. It is yellow-red in color with scalloped-edge. It is usually unilateral and does not metastasize. In most cases are asymptomatic but approximately 30% to 50% of patients will eventually develop choroidal neovascularization leading to visual loss [16, 17]. Differential diagnosis includes amelanotic choroidal melanoma and choroidal metastases. Choroidal osteoma in the FA shows early hypofluorescence with slow enhancement thereof.

The presence of inconspicuous hypofluorescent spicules on their surface is very characteristic of this tumor. Using A-mode ultrasound, there is a large initial peak product of the high internal reflectivity of the tumor. On B-mode ultrasound an echogenic dense calcium plaque followed by an acoustic shadowing is a characteristic pattern of choroidal osteoma [18].

5. Choroidal Metastasis

Metastases are the most common malignant intraocular tumors in adulthood. They are usually located in the posterior pole and can be solitary or multiple lesions. The bilateral involvement is also common. Metastatic lesions can be flat either dome-shaped appearance, thus in this case they can be confused with an amelanotic melanoma. The primary tumors most frequently involved in metastatic ocular disease are: the lung in men and breast cancer in women. When metastases occur in the choroid, the tumor is usually at an advanced stage therefore with a poor clinically prognosis for these patients. The Choroidal metastasis are usually diagnosed by incidental or also because the visual impairment they produce. The macula may be affected by direct tumor infiltration or also by the presence of exudative retinal detachment. The FA shows an early hypofluorescence and diffuse late-phase hyperfluorescence. Ocular ultrasound B-mode shows the solid character of the metastatic lesions (Fig. **4**). Retinal detachment is a very common finding. Unlike regmatogenous retinal detachment, subretinal fluid varies with the movements of the head [19]. In the A-mode ultrasound, the internal reflectivity is mild throughout the tumor, which is indicative but not pathognomonic for choroidal metastases.

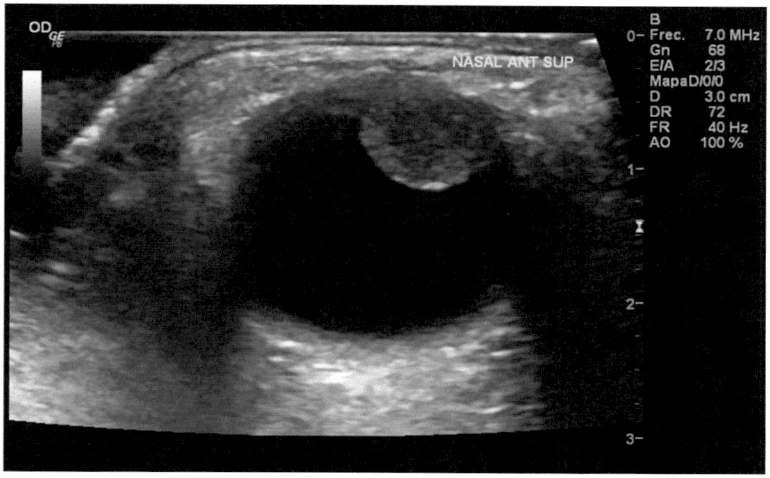

Figure 4: Metastasis of mama carcinoma, in superior quadrant, close to the ciliar body.

RETINA

1. Retinoblastoma

It is the most common intraocular tumor of childhood. It may be sporadic or familiar. As it presents as a leukocoria, the differential diagnosis with familial exudative vitreoretinopathy, retinopathy of prematurity, persistent hyperplastic primary vitreous and Coats disease must be made. The ocular ultrasound is the most efficient test for the differential diagnosis of leukocoria. In the presence of a retinoblastoma, the ultrasound shows a tumor with endophytic growth and typical hyperechoic intratumoral calcifications [20, 21].

OPTIC NERVE

1. Capillary Hemangioma of the Optic Nerve

The capillary hemangioma of the optic disc is a benign tumor of vascular nature. It can occur in isolation or as part of the Von Hippel-Lindau syndrome. The capillary hemangioma appears as a raised rosy lesion in the optic nerve head. Perilesional lipid exudation may occur, and when this happens the macula is often affected by proximity, resulting in a significant visual loss. Again, the FA and ocular ultrasound are the most useful complementary tests for the study of this tumor. At FA we observe angiographic hyperfluorescence in early times that last until later times. At this stage appears suffusion of the fluorescein, suggesting the vascular nature of the tumor. In A-mode ocular ultrasound, there is a high initial reflectivity peak with a subsequent decrease on it. In B-mode ocular ultrasound, there is a small homogeneous lesion in the optic nerve head, often accompanied by perilesional retinal detachment with macular involvement. Color-Doppler ultrasound reveals the hypervascularity of the tumor.

2. Optic Nerve Melanocytoma

It is a benign tumor that is observed on the optic nerve head [22]. It's a pigmented lesion that extends to peripapillary area. Most times it is congenital, usually stationary or slow growing and no association with systemic diseases has been found. The assessment by FA shows a pattern of relatively hypofluorescence. By A-mode ultrasound melanocytomas usually show medium or high internal reflectivity (Fig. **5**). Color-Doppler echography reveals the absence of tumor vascularization [23]. If thickness increased or vascularization is detected, a melanoma transformation must be suspected.

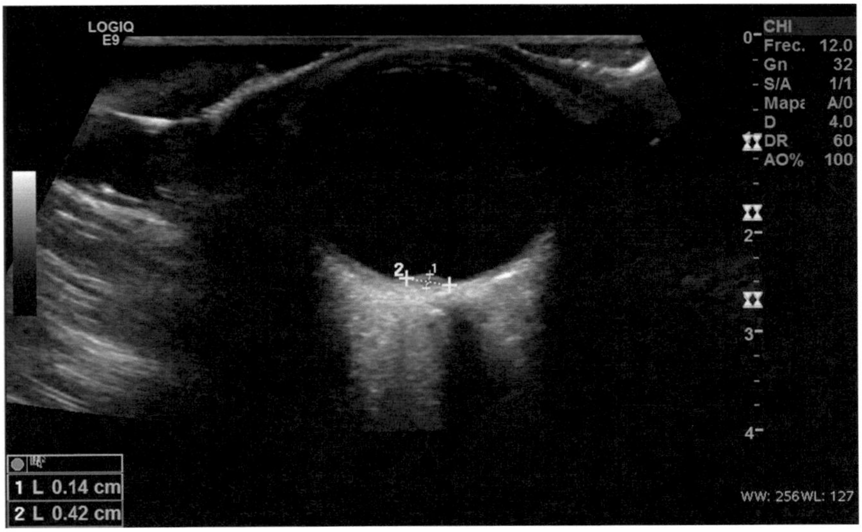

Figure 5: Melanocitoma of papilla, size 0.14 x 0.42 cm.

CONCLUDING REMARKS

The intraocular tumors are the most important pathologies which ultrasounds examinations are applied. The echography is basic for choroid melanoma diagnosis, currently the ultrasounds are the first technique used in melanoma suspect. Furthermore the differential diagnosis between melanoma and other tumors as carcinoma metastasis is based in echography findings.

ACKNOWLEDGEMENTS

Declared None.

CONFLICT OF INTEREST

The authors confirm that this chapter contents have no conflict of interest.

REFERENCES

[1] Sullivan TJ, Clarke MP, Morin JD. The ocular manifestations of the Sturge-Weber syndrome. J Pediatr Ophthalmol Strabismus. 1992, 29: 349-56.

[2] Mashayekhi A, Shields CL. Circumscribed choroidal hemangioma. Curr Opin Ophthalmol. 2003, 14(3): 142-9.

[3] Anand R, Augsburger JJ, Shields JA. Circumscribed choroidal hemangiomas. Arch Ophthalmol. 1989, 107: 1338-42.

[4] Ingh A, Kaiser P, Sears J. Choroidal hemangioma. Ophthalmol Clin North Am 2005 18: 151-61.

[5] Sumich P, Mitchell P, Wang JJ. Choroidal nevi in a white population: The Blue Mountains Eye Study. Arch Ophthalmol. 1998, 116(5): 645-650.
[6] Aiserman I, Kaiserman N, Pe'er J. Long term ultrasonic follow up of choroidal naevi and their transformation to melanomas Br J Ophthalmol 2006, 90: 994-8.
[7] Desjardins L, Lumbroso L, Levy C, *et al.* Facteurs of risque pour la dégénérescence des naevi choroïdiens: étude sur rétrospective 135 cas J Fr Ophthalmol 2001, 24: 610-6.
[8] August. G, Espinoza, Rosenblatt B, *et al.* Optical coherence tomography in the evaluation of retinal changes Associated with suspicious choroidal melanocytic tumors Am J Ophthalmol 2004, 137: 90-5.
[9] Hields CL, Cater J, Shields JA, *et al.* Combination of clinical factors predictive of growth of small choroidal melanocytic tumors Arch Ophthalmol 2000, 118: 360-4.
[10] Carol L, Shields, Minoru F, *et al.* Shields. Choroidal nevus transformation into melanoma. Analysis of 2514 consecutive cases. Arch Ophthalmol. 2009, 127(8): 981-7.
[11] The Collaborative Ocular Melanoma Study(COMS) randomized trial of pre-enucleation radiation of large choroidal melanoma II: initial mortality findings. COMS report No. 10. Am J Ophthalmol. 1998, 125: 779-96.
[12] Mooy CM, De Jong PT. Prognostic parameters in uveal melanoma: a review. Surv Ophthalmol. 1996, 41: 215-28.
[13] JD Coleman. Echography of eye and orbit. 2nd ed. Lippincott: Williams and Wilkins, pp. 47-122.
[14] John A. The eye and orbit, Fielding. In: Cosgrove D, editor. Clinical Ultrasound. 2001. pp. 659-95. Parson's T / B of Diseases of Eye. 19th ed. Elsevier, 2003.
[15] Gass JD, Guerry RK, Jack RL, *et al.* Choroidal osteoma. Arch Ophthalmol. 1978, 96: 428-35.
[16] Aylward GW, Chang TS, Pautler SE, *et al.* A long-term follow-up of choroidal osteoma. Arch Ophthalmol. 1998, 116: 1337-41.
[17] Kadrmas EF, Weiter JJ. Choroidal osteoma. Int Ophthalmol Clin. 1997 37: 171-82.
[18] Tost F, Schmidt U. Electrophysiologic and echographic findings with choroidal osteoma. Ophthalmologica. 1998, 212(6): 377-80.
[19] Freedman MI, Folk JC. Metastatic tumors to the eye and orbit: patient survival and clinical characteristics. Arch Ophthalmol 1987, 105: 1216-9.
[20] Coleman JD. Echography of eye and orbit. 2nd ed. Lippincott: Williams and Wilkins, pp. 47-122.
[21] John A. The eye and orbit, Fielding. In: Cosgrove D, editor. Clinical Ultrasound. 2001; 659-95.
[22] Joffe L, Shields JA, Osher RH, *et al.* Clinical and follow-up studies of melanocytomas of the optic disc. Ophthalmology. 1979, 86(6): 1067-1083.
[23] Di Bernardo C, Pacheco EM, Hughes JR, *et al.* Echographic evaluation and findings in metastatic melanoma to extraocular muscles. Ophthalmology. 1996, 103(11): 1794-7.

CHAPTER 6

Color-Doppler Eye Scan Ultrasound

Manuel Montero-Jaime[1,*], Pedro Romero-Aroca[2,*] and Javier Reyes-Torres[2]

[1]*Department of Radiology* [2], *Department of Ophthalmology, University Hospital Sant Joan, Rovira & Virgili University, Pere Virgili Health Research Institute, IISPV, Reus, Spain*

Abstract: The Color-Doppler ultrasound introduced a new point of view in all ocular vasculopathies, thus the diabetic retinopathy [DR] can be studied based in the alterations in the ocular flux, currently DR is studied by scanning laser system, but this technique only permit us to view the intra retinal flux changes, but not the changes which succeed in choroid or in retro ocular vessels, which Color-Doppler ultrasound permit us to observe with an easy noninvasive examination. Furthermore the Color-Doppler echography is useful in patients with a decrease of vascular flux due to carotid insufficiency. Other pathologies as intraocular venous occlusions or arterial embolism produce typical signs in Color-Doppler echography. In this chapter we describe the basis of Color-Doppler examination for ocular vessels, the normal values for each vessel [ophthalmic artery or veins, central artery and vein, and for ciliary vessels], and the typical alterations observed in each vascular pathology.

Keywords: Color-Doppler ultrasound, diabetic retinopathy, central artery occlusions, venous retinal occlusions, anterior segment ischemia, posterior segment ischemia.

INTRODUCTION

Color-Doppler ultrasound study of the ocular vascularization has proven its utility in various entities. The principle of measuring the velocity of an object by using the shift of frequency of two light or sound waves [in our case, the use of ultrasound] was first described by Christian Andreas Doppler in the nineteenth century. The application of the Color-Doppler principle [as is now known] to ultrasound dates back to 1957, and it is established as a routine method of clinical research of the large blood vessels in the body. In recent years, its use has been expanded to the study of smaller size vessels being introduced to the study of blood flow velocity in orbital vessels by Erickson [1], Lieb *et al.*, [2] and Baxter *et al.*, [3]. By using ocular Color-Doppler ultrasound, the studied blood vessels overlap on a B-mode ultrasound.

***Corresponding author Manuel Montero-Jaime:** Hospital Universitario Sant Joan, Avda. Doctor Josep Laporte 1 Reus, Spain; E-mail: mmontero@grupsagessa.com
Pedro Romero Aroca: Hospital Universitario Sant Joan, Avda. Doctor Josep Laporte 1 Reus, Spain; E-mail: pormero@grupsagessa.com

INDICATIONS

The indications of ocular Color-Doppler ultrasound study include the study of the following vessels: ophthalmic artery and vein, posterior ciliary arteries, central retinal artery and vein (Table **1**).

Table 1: Color-Doppler echography, indications

Ocular tumors	
Ocular vascular pathology	➢ Central retinal vein occlusion ➢ Central retinal artery occlusion ➢ Chronic retinal ischemia [carotid insufficiency] ➢ Glaucoma ➢ Diabetic retinopathy ➢ Retinal detachment [tractional RD differential diagnosis] ➢ Optic neuropathy ➢ Vascular origin [Horton's disease, non-arteritic ischemic optic neuropathy] ➢ Inflammatory origin [Multiple sclerosis, sarcoidosis, *etc.*] ➢ Papillary tumors [hemangioma]
Orbital masses	➢ Vascularized [capillary angiomas *etc.*] ➢ Hypervascularized [Cavernous hemangioma, mixed tumor of the lacrimal gland] ➢ Non-vascularized cysts
Carotid-cavernous fistula	

OBTAINED MEASUREMENTS

There are only used a series of blood flow velocity indicators from the Color-Doppler ultrasound obtained pulse wave [1-4].

1. Blood Flow Measurements

The measures will differ depending on the target vessel, and the blood flow study includes the determination of:

- Peak systolic flow velocity [PSV]
- Peak diastolic flow velocity [EDV]
- Arterial resistance index [ARI] or Pourcelot index
- Artery pulsatility index is calculated by the formula [API]

The formulas to obtain the resistance index and pulse rate are:

1. Arterial resistance index [ARI] or Pourcelot index= [PSV-EDV]/PSV

2. Artery pulsatility index [API] = [PSV-EDV]/Tmax Acronim: Tmax = the average time of peak velocity

3. *Venous flow measurements*

For its part, the venous flow study includes the determination of:

- Maximum speed [Vmax]

- Minimum speed [V min]

- Venous pulsatility index [IPV] or Gosling index

The formula for venous pulsatility index rate is: VPI = [Vmax-Vmin]/Vmin

The determination of the flow velocity, as observed in the preferred measurement of venous flow characteristics, is that the observed flow wave is more uniform making it difficult to determine velocity peaks. The resistance index [known as Pourcelot' ratio] is scored from 0% to 100% [0 to 1 cm/sec, depending on the type of dimming] representing 0% no resistance and 100% maximum resistance to the blood flow. As we will see in front of all the parameters quoted before, the resistance index is the one that has a higher value in the clinical study of blood vessels. The resistance index is intended to be measured in the arterial vessels [central retinal ophthalmic artery], while the pulsating rate is better as measure rate of venous vessels. The average values, for each parameter, are shown in Table **2** [3-10]. The reproducibility of these values is greater when the observed values are higher, and for the obtained values in the small ocular blood vessels are smaller; because the detection equipment used affect the determination of such securities. If the used equipment determines values between 1 and 3 cm/sec, we will see lack of flow in small vessels, by giving a wrong picture of vessel closure, when this does not exist, and it is a determination defect of the equipment, by stating, only, that the flow values are in the determination limit of the used instrument.

Table 2: Normal values of different flow parameters

	Ophthalmic artery	Central retinal artery	Posterior ciliary arteries
Systolic velocity peak [PSV]	26,34-33,27 cm/sec	5,56-8,58 cm/sec	8,90-14,18 cm/sec
Diastolic velocity peak [EDV]	2,85-6,81 cm/sec	1,51-2,85 cm/sec	1,85-3,69 cm/sec
Resistance index	83,0% [0,83]	70% [0,70]	65 % [0,65]

2. Angle Measurement Effect in the Flow Values Determination

The Doppler Effect is used to calculate the blood cells' passing speed through the vessel thanks to the frequency change of ultrasound reflected on them. The larger the Doppler shift is in frequency, the faster the cells will be. However, the observed change depends, largely, on the emitted ultrasound beam is parallel to the blood flow, and if the beam is not parallel to the flow, the observed change will be less. The required angle that causes a significant error in flow velocity is high, generally above 45 degrees. In ocular vessels and orbit flow determination, we can observe that the flow follows an antero-posterior direction, so the angle of incidence is low. However in order to avoid errors, the determination of the resistance index is the less influenced value by these changes, because is integrated the error caused by a change of angle of incidence, as this rate is a ratio and not a peak speed.

OCULAR AND ORBITAL BLOOD VESSELS EXAM

1. Examination Technique

In general, it is necessary to make, by first, a type B ultrasound examination of the ocular globe and to locate the optic nerve, prior to the Color-Doppler scanning. Put the patient in supine position with the eyes closed and using an ultrasound frequency higher than 7 MHz and a Doppler frequency higher than 5 MHz. The transducer is applied on top over the upper eyelid using a layer of acoustic gel and placing the examiner hand on the orbital margin to minimize the pressure on the ocular globe, which it will alter the blood flow measurement outcome, especially on the diastolic velocity values with the resulting increase of resistance index. Color-Doppler echography is performed by the settled gain so that avoids noisy artifacts in color, by allowing the detection of lower speeds. Then, the tip of the Doppler [<2mm] is placed on the detected vessel in order to obtain the blood flow signals. Although as is previously mentioned, the ocular and orbital blood vessels are parallel to the ultrasound beam; you can use a correction angle, as described above, in cases where required. We will use the lower frequency probe that will allow us a good spatial resolution in B-mode, typically 9 MHz, both with color and pulsed Doppler we obtain information about the vessels presence, and direction and characteristics of flow. The power Doppler is sensitive to slower flow and useful for newvesels detection. During Color-Doppler examination, we will obtain information about the ophthalmic artery, the central retinal artery and vein, and the posterior ciliary arteries. The ophthalmic artery will be easy to locate medial to the optic nerve, by showing a relatively high resistance wave morphology with normal systolic velocities of 31.4 +/-4.2 cm/sec [2]. The central retinal vessels are jointly explored by its close proximity relationship, by appearing the artery with a wave of low resistance, that is rounded peak systolic and positive diastole. The average speed is 10.3 cm/sec [9] while the vein shows a continuous flow in the opposite direction to the artery with speeds of 3 cm/sec. The posterior ciliary arteries will be identified in the posterior fat of the ocular globe, on both sides of the optic nerve, with a low resistance pattern and average speeds of 12 cm/sec.

LOCATION OF THE VESSELS

Firstly, there must get a B-mode ultrasound of the eye locating the optic nerve, which is located medial to the orbit (Fig. **1**). Then, we must proceed to locate the vessel that we want to study:

1. Ophthalmic Artery and Veins

Ophthalmic vessels are found behind the ocular globe, and they are located in flat and slightly above the optic nerve (Fig. **2**). The vascular waveform of the ophthalmic artery is similar to the one of the internal carotid artery, with an elevated systolic peak [PSV], followed by a rapid descent to the diastolic peak [EDV]. It can be seen, in this descending, a notch in midway coinciding with the aortic valve closure. The ophthalmic vein location would be adjacent to the artery. The blood velocity in the ophthalmic artery varies with age, systemic blood pressure, smoking, and possibly, in the same manner, by depending on the subject position. The angle determination in respect of the ultrasound beam is easy to determine, and it can help us to extrapolate the results obtained to other measurements. It is important that the patient stays with its eyes still and directed to the position recommended by the browser. The results obtained in the nasal portion of the orbit are usually detected better, but unfortunately in this position the central retinal vessels and the ciliary vessels have already left the ophthalmic artery, which much of the information is lost; thus, we recommend detecting the blood flow information in the vascular portion located on the optic or temporal nerve at the same.

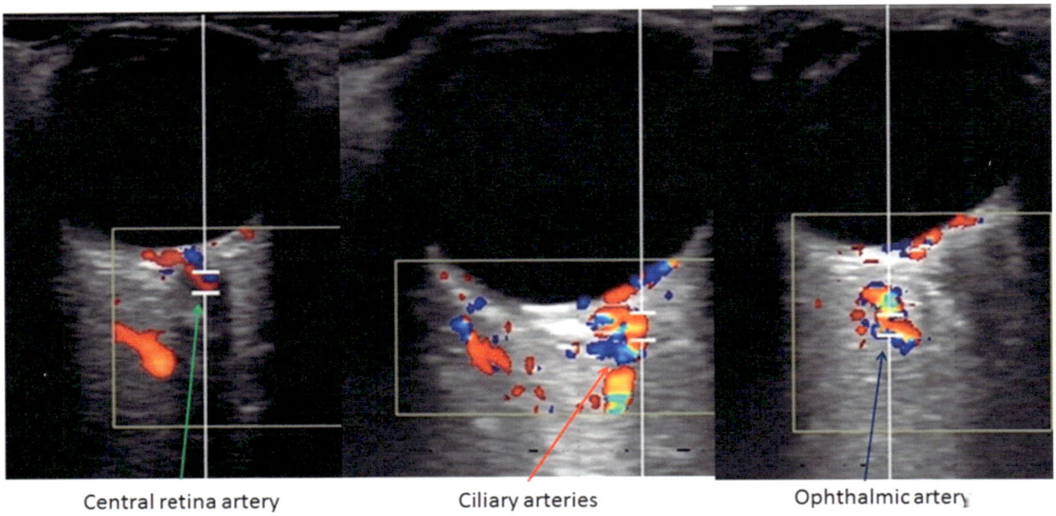

Figure 1: Color doppler of ocular vessels, location where we encountered the maximum activity.

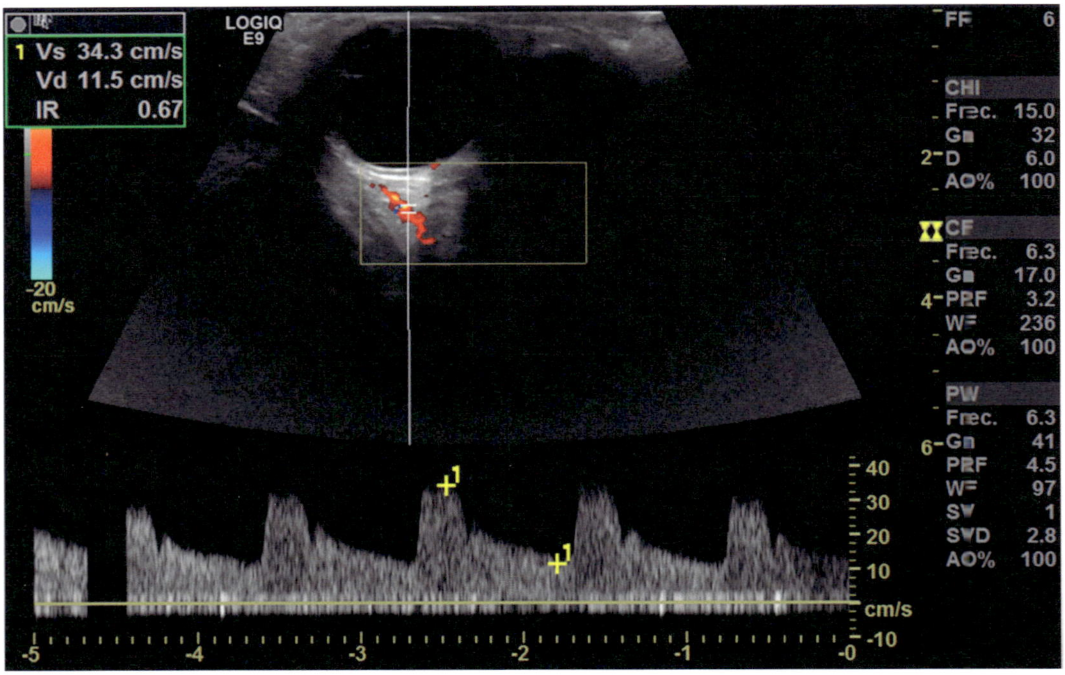

Figure 2: Color doppler of ophthalmic artery. In the box on the left are the observed values.

2. Central Retina Artery and Vein Vessels

They can be detected inside the optic nerve, in the retro-laminar portion, along of 10 mm length immediately behind the ocular globe. The vein is located immediately adjacent to the artery, while the artery is on the nasal side, and the vein is on the temporal side (Fig. **3**); it is observed as a blue band, and another one red, inside the optic nerve, and it forms an angle of about 15 degrees to the antero-posterior axis. The wave produced by the central retinal artery is clearly inferior to the one of the ophthalmic artery. At the central retinal vessels level, we can get all the usual parameters values of the vascular flow study [PSV, EDV, pulsatility index, resistance index].

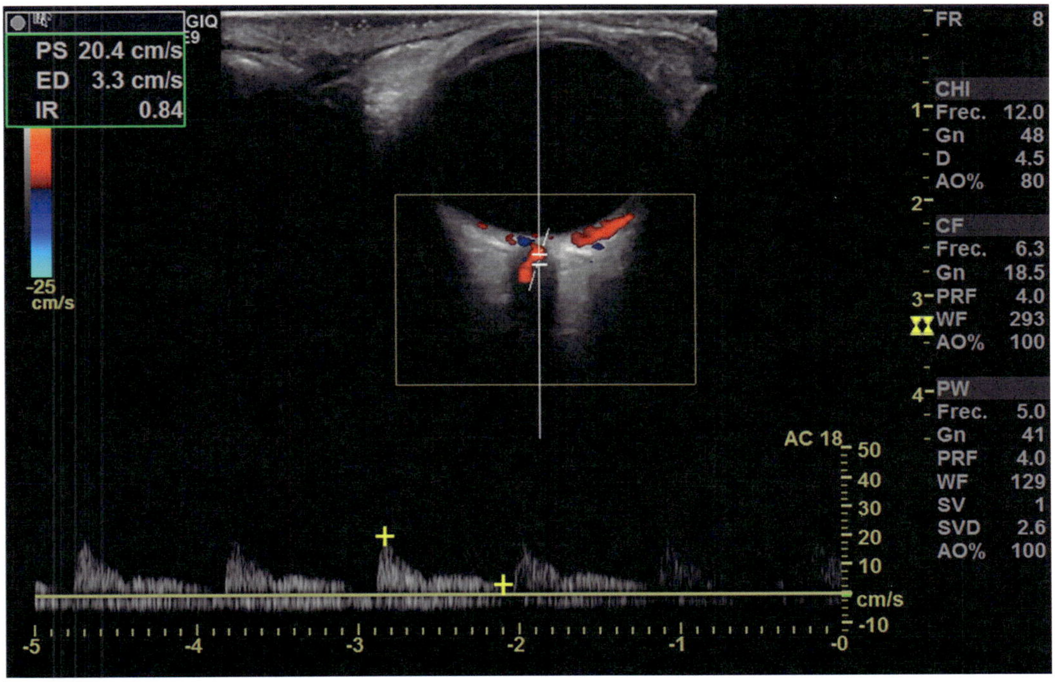

Figure 3: Color doppler of central artery.

3. Posterior Ciliary Vessels

It forms a series of vascular trunks approximately located from 10 to 20 mm behind the ocular globe and surrounds the optic nerve in its retrobulbar portion. The obtained vascular waveform is similar to those of the central retinal vessels, but with a more pronounced diastolic peak. Its examination has to be done in the nasal and temporal regions of the optic nerve (Fig. **4**). The differentiation between the two types of the existing ciliary vessels [long and short posterior] is difficult and rarely achieved. It is hard to know the number of ciliary vessels by ranging in number from one individual to another therefore it is difficult to know how many vessels are being studied using Color-Doppler ultrasound [7-9]. The measuring results in the retro-orbital portion is the least reproducible due to the high tortuosity of these vessels in the area; it is recommended the study of ciliary vessels in the peri-laminar portion [near of the optic nerve's entrance to the ocular globe]. Of all the vascular parameters, the resistance index, which is independent of the angle formed by the ultrasound beam, is the most reproducible parameter and therefore the one that must be determined when these blood vessels are explored. An important fact to keep in mind is that blood flow at the level of the ciliary vessels is highly dependent of intraocular pressure, so we must avoid putting pressure on the ocular globe at the moment of exploring the ciliary vessels.

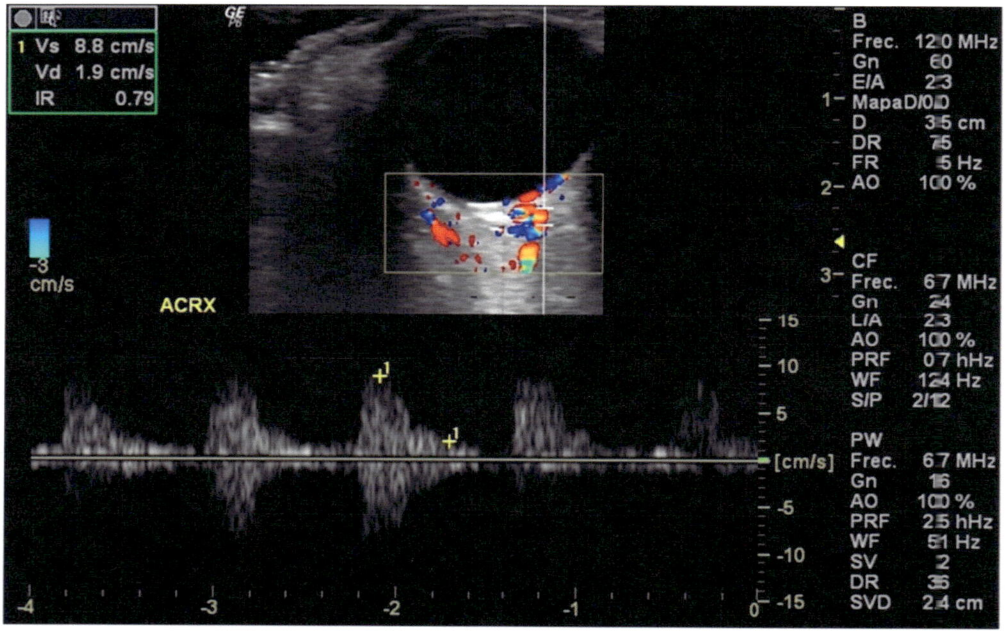

Figure 4: Color doppler of ciliary arteries.

4. Vorticose Veins

They are located in the horizontal plane above and below of the optic nerve plane, and exactly placed in the ocular globe equator, by showing the type of constant velocity venous flow.

5. Superior Ophthalmic Vein

The ophthalmic vein is divided into two parts, an upper one and a lower one; the

MEASURES INTERPRETATION

First of all, we must say that the values determined by Color-Doppler ultrasound are blood velocity measurements and not of flow. The flow would be the result from the following formula:

$$F = V \times \pi r\ 2$$

Acronyms: F = flow, V = velocity, r = radius

The interpretation of the blood velocity results obtained, as a measure of blood perfusion of the studied tissues, is purely speculative because we ignore the vessel diameter, measure that cannot be determined with ultrasound and may be misleading. So, if there is any vascular stenosis, the speed may be increased, but total blood flow could be decreased. In any case, the resistance index and the pulsatility index measuring are the two most important and reproducible measures in Color-Doppler ultrasound because these report to us a fairly reliable estimate about the state of the explored vessel blood flow, so when the blood flow resistance grows in a determined vessel, these two indexes values significantly grows.

VASCULAR OCCLUSIONS

1. Ophthalmic and Internal Carotid Artery Stenosis

In case of a chronic hypoperfusion of the ophthalmic artery, we will have to suspect that its origin is, mostly often, at the level of the carotid artery, secondary to a stenosis of it. Several studies have shown a blood velocity drop of the central retinal artery, if the carotid artery stenosis is greater than 70%. The clinical picture that we will observe is of an anterior ischemia syndrome; it is visible at the fundus of the eye level with shapes of round hemorrhages and isolated on the temporal side. The patient will present a progressive loss of vision, and in advanced cases it may appear neovascular glaucoma secondary to the ischemia. If an endarterectomy is effectively performed, we would be able to see the ocular signs disappearance and a bigger ocular perfusion on Doppler ultrasound of the ophthalmic artery and its branches.

2. Central Retinal Artery Occlusion

The central retinal artery occlusion can be easily diagnosed by fundus examination, but if there is any opacity in the media, the Color-Doppler ultrasound may be useful. In the acute phase, it can be observed an absence of the Doppler signal at the optic nerve level, by not observing the typical arterial waveform image, equally the venous flow, and thus the venous wave image is diminished. The arterial recanalization happens soon, within the first or second week after occlusion, and showing a return to normality in the arterial and venous ultrasound waves [11].

3. Central Retinal Vein Occlusion

There is a marked decrease in venous blood velocity in patients who have suffered a central retinal vein occlusion; with decreased venous wave, we can easily verify this fact by observing the normal venous wave in the contralateral eye. There are differences between the central retinal vein edematous occlusion and the ischemic forms; also there are differences if the occlusion affects only one branch of the central vein. In case of branch retinal vein occlusion, the flow rate may be normal and not been observed abnormalities in the venous parameters, especially the pulsatility index. In case of central retinal vein edematous occlusion, it can be seen, according to some authors [12], an increase in the resistance index, although some other authors have not found this as significant [3]. Arai *et al.,* [13] have demonstrated that the presence of a low minimum speed is the predictor of a retinal vascular ischemia associated with the vein occlusion. Thus, the presence of a minimum venous initial velocity lower than 3 cm/sec has been shown to be a neovascularization risk sign at the level of iris [3]. The presence of a high resistance index is associated with low acuity in patients. Finally, the parameters study of the central retinal artery show that it remains in normal levels, by demonstrating that the occlusion affects only to the central retinal vein.

4. Ischemic Optic Neuropathies

The ischemic optic neuropathies can be classified into two groups:

- Arteritic [AION] or Horton disease
- Non-arteritic [NOIN], secondary to vascular diseases such as diabetic retinopathy or arterial hypertension, or more often a combination of both

In the cranial arteritis [Horton's arteritis], it can be seen that the flow, at the ophthalmic artery level, is almost undetectable even if the patient's general condition suggests that is recovering from the process, by giving the image of an empty socket, since we cannot detect signs of vascular risk in all orbital or ocular vessels. We will observe changes in vascular parameters, especially a decline in the systolic peak and an increase of the resistance index at the level of various ocular arteries. So in Ghanchi *et al.,* [14] study on 7 patients with Horton's arteritis, it were observed alterations in the central retinal artery, posterior ciliary arteries and ophthalmic artery in 6 patients, and after the management through medication of the arteritic incident, it showed the parameters normalization in 4 patients who recovered normal vision and remaining with low vision the other two. The non-arteritic ischemic optic neuropathies are the most common by far, and they occur in elderly patients; these are the occlusion or hypoperfusion result of the optic nerve papilla from the posterior ciliary arteries. The diagnosis is mainly clinical and includes: visual acuity loss, altitudinal visual field defects, color vision defects [red-green axis involvement] and sectorial papilledema. When a Color-Doppler ultrasound is performed in these patients, we observe a decreased systolic peak and an increased resistance index at the posterior ciliary arteries level; also in some cases, you can see the same signs at the central retinal artery level, but with changes much less pronounced, since the main lesion is located at the posterior ciliary level [4]. Once the occlusion episode has spontaneously disappeared, the altered values are normalized.

TUMORS

The intraocular tumors exploration with Color-Doppler ultrasound can be helpful to achieve a proper diagnosis; the presence of intraocular masses is easily to determine with B-mode ultrasound, and, in fact, it is important its use for a proper diagnosis of choroid melanomas due to the typical image of the same in the B-mode ultrasound. Also, the Color-Doppler ultrasound will be of great help for determining the presence of intratumoral vascularization, especially in highly vascularized tumors [1].

1. Choroid Hemangiomas

The high vascularization of these tumors allows to perform a Color-Doppler ultrasound and to observe the great blood velocity in them, by clearly differentiating it from the choroid melanomas, which are tumors that in the echography have similar characteristics.

2. Papillary Tumors

The provided information in these tumors, by fluorescein angiography, is superior to Color-Doppler ultrasound information, but this latter technique allows us to provide information about other effects produced by the tumor itself, as compression on adjacent structures such as the papilla, the retina or the choroid.

PSEUDOTUMORS

Sometimes patients with age-related macular degeneration, in its neovascular form, present images of notable growth of the lesion giving a pseudotumoral image; this is hard to distinguish from other tumors such as choroid melanoma. The practice of Color-Doppler ultrasound in these patients may help in observing a significant internal vascularization in the pseudotumor AMD, in front of other tumors such as choroid melanoma, tumor that we always have to keep in mind in the differential diagnosis of tumor masses in the fundus of the eye.

DIABETIC RETINOPATHY

The diabetic retinopathy, as we have described in another chapter, is one of the leading causes of blindness in the western world, with an expected increase of diabetic patients in the coming years; it becomes a major health problem. The proper diagnosis of the ocular involvement in the diabetic allows a better control over it and a decreasing in the number of blind patients. One of the imaging techniques used in the diagnosis of injuries caused by diabetic retinopathy includes B-mode ultrasound, as described in the previous chapter, besides the Color-Doppler ultrasound can provide us significant information for the diagnosis and treatment of the diabetic patient's complications. The systolic peak velocity is decreased in patients with diabetic retinopathy. Thus, Goebel *et al.,* [15] found an average PSV of 8.4 ± 1.8 cm/sec in patients with nonproliferative retinopathy, and an average PSV of 5.7 ± 1 8 cm/sec in those with proliferative retinopathy; in opposition to normal of average PSV of 9.4 ± 1.2 cm/sec in the control group. It is common that media opacities exist in diabetic patients, as the presence of cataract or vitreous hemorrhage. In the first case, the practice of a B-mode ultrasound will allows us to exclude the presence of a vitreous hemorrhage or a tractional retinal detachment in these eligible patients for cataract surgery, by giving us the basic information to set the surgery type to perform. Additionally, the performing of a Doppler ultrasound in the same can give us that necessary information to know what we will find during surgery [16, 17]. So, it is important to determine the presence of new-vessels at retinal or papillary level. In the diagnosis of proliferative diabetic retinopathy, we will locate them above the papilla of the optic nerve or the equator globe at the vascular arcades level. Recently, the Color-Doppler ultrasound has been useful for the diagnosis of a recent knowledge entity, the formation of new-vessels at the sclerotomies of entry level during the practice of posterior vitrectomy. It is recognized that the presence of these new-vessels is the most common cause of hemorrhage after a posterior vitrectomy practice, which is important its recognition for its treatment in order to avoid a new hemorrhage that would lead to multiple vitreous surgeries.

GLAUCOMA

The primary open-angle glaucoma is, by far, the most common form of glaucoma in the population; it is considered to be an optic neuropathy that has a multifactorial origin. Although, the growth of intraocular pressure is the most important known cause of optic nerve damage, other factors are involved in its pathogenesis. Lately, the perfusion of the optic nerve intraocular portion has attracted attention, and various techniques have been proposed to investigate the circulation hemodynamics at the optic nerve level. The measurement of several quantitative parameters has attracted interest to evaluate the hemodynamic changes and to assess whether these are from primary cause of glaucomatous neuropathy or are secondary to it. The advantage of Color-Doppler ultrasound, in this condition, is that it allows us to assess in real-time the blood flow at the retrobulbar region.

1. Study of Flow Parameters Changes

The significance of the observed changes at the ocular blood flow level is difficult to analyze. Thus, a decrease in the diastolic peak is an indication of vascular impedance increase that will lead to a vascular resistance index increase. The increase of vascular resistance will affect to a greater extent the systolic flow rather than the diastolic flow. In the published studies, it is shown that there is an increase in the resistance index of the vessels located around the intraocular portion of the optic nerve in glaucoma patients; the increase of the intraocular pressure, the vasoconstriction, the vasospasm, and other several factors have been recognized as potential coadjuvant to increase vascular resistance. According to various authors [9-11], the chronic growth of the intraocular pressure would be the most important factor to produce the observed hemodynamic changes. On the contrary, the changes observed at the ophthalmic artery level could be to an increase of PCO_2, by indicating that it would be originated from a possible vasospasm, especially in a subgroup of patients as those with normal tension glaucoma.

An interesting fact, which is observed in published studies, is that the peak systolic velocity [PSV] is increased in some patients without prior treatment [12]. Now, since the diastolic peak is decreased and the resistance index is increased; there has been speculated with the possibility of that the PSV is increased to compensate the decrease of the blood flow, which the parameters mentioned above behaves. Finally, we must consider the study of Trible *et al.,* [18] that shows an improvement of vascular parameters after the trabeculectomy performing and the return of the intraocular pressure back to normal levels.

2. Changes Observed at the Level of the Central Retinal Artery and the Posterior Ciliary

Various studies have been prepared about the blood vascularization by Color-Doppler ultrasound. Most of the patients with chronic open-angle glaucoma, especially in its variation of normal-tension glaucoma, have shown that the diastolic peak [EDV] is decreased, and the resistance index is elevated; both at the level of the central retinal artery and the posterior ciliary arteries. Also, it has been found a decrease in the systolic peak [PSV] in some studies, but this decline is less pronounced than the EDV values [11].

3. Changes Observed at the Ophthalmic Artery Level

The findings at the level of the ophthalmic artery are more complex. Thus, although the diastolic peak [EDV] is decreased in the majority of the studies, the disparity is present in relation with the systolic peak [PSV]; some authors have shown the decline of such values, but instead UVT *et al.,* have found higher values than the normal for PSV. Likewise, Kayser *et al.,* [12] have not found significant changes of the same parameter in patients after the use of antiglaucoma medications.

4. Relationship between Visual Field and Doppler Ultrasound

One of the basic examinations in the diagnosis of glaucoma is the practice of a visual field; currently, the standard technique is the one performed by Humphrey automated perimetry. The presence of typical visual field defects of glaucoma [such as nasal step or arcuate scotomas] gives the necessary information for a proper diagnosis and, also, for a proper tracking of glaucoma patients. Therefore, it is important the correlation between the observed changes in the visual field resulting from the damage at the optic nerve level and the hemodynamic changes observed by Color-Doppler ultrasound. In fact, several studies have shown that hemodynamic changes are associated and even preceded to visual field alterations. So, Rankin [19] found an association between visual field loss and a decrease of the peak diastolic velocity [EDV]. Equally, a study in a group of patients with asymmetric glaucoma, in which one eye was more affected than the contralateral, noticed that the peaks diastolic velocity were diminished, and the resistance index were increased in both eyes; although, the visual field defects are observed just in one of them, this finding may indicate that hemodynamic changes precede to glaucoma's visual field injuries.

CONCLUDING REMARKS

We have to keep in mind that Color-Doppler ultrasound gives us values about the velocity of blood flow, but it does not measure the blood flow itself because we should have the knowledge of the vascular diameter, which it does not determine the ultrasound *per se*. Despite of this limitation, the determination of the flow velocity gives us important information about blood flow in itself. So that, we can consider that the observed changes, about the hemodynamic in patients with glaucoma, can be an important factor in the damage at the optic nerve level observed in these patients. Although, these changes may be secondary to the increase of the intraocular pressure in some patients; in other, the vascular factor would be the origin of them.

ACKNOWLEDGEMENTS

Declared None.

CONFLICT OF INTEREST

The authors confirm that this chapter contents have no conflict of interest.

REFERENCES

[1] Erickson SJ, Hendrix LE, Massaro BM, *et al.* Color-Doppler flow imaging of the normal and abnormal orbit. Radiology 1989; 173: 511.
[2] Lieb WE. Color-Doppler imaging of the eye and orbit. Radiol Clin North Am 1998; 36: 1059.
[3] Baxter GM, Williamson TH. Color-Doppler flow imaging in central retinal vein occlusion: a new diagnostic technique? Radiology 1993; 187: 847.
[4] Braband K, Kerty E, Jakobsen JA. Contrast enhanced ultrasound Doppler examination of the retrobulbar arteries. Acta Radiol 2001; 42: 135.
[5] Berger RW, Guthoff R, Helmke K, *et al.* Colorcoded Doppler echography of orbital blood vessels with special reference to the central retinal artery and vein. Fortschr Ophthalmol 1991; 88: 690.

[6] Guthoff RF, Berger RW, Winkler P, *et al.* Doppler echography of the ophthalmic and central retinal vessels. Arch Ophthalmol 1991; 109: 532.

[7] Harris A, Kagemann L, Cioffi G. Assessment of human ocular hemodynamics. Surv Ophthalmol 1998; 42: 509.

[8] Kaiser HJ, Shötzau A, Stümpfig D, *et al.* Blood flow velocities of the extraocular vessels in patients with high-tension and normal-tension primary open-angle glaucoma. Am J Ophthalmol 1997; 123: 320.

[9] Lieb WE, Flaharty PM, Ho A, *et al.* Color-Doppler imaging of the eye and orbit. A synopsis of a 400-case experience. Acta Ophthalmol 1992; 204: 50.

[10] Williamson TH, Baxter GM, Pyott A, *et al.* A comparison of Color-Doppler imaging of orbital vessels and other methods of blood flow assessment. Graefes Arch Clin Exp Ophthalmol 1995; 233: 80.

[11] Guthoff RF, Berger RW, Winkler P, *et al.* Doppler echography of the ophthalmic and central retinal vessels. Arch Ophthalmol 1991; 109: 532.

[12] Senn BC, Kaiser HJ, Schötzau A, Flammer J. Reproducibility of color Doppler imaging in orbital vessels. Ger J Ophthalmol. 1996; 5(6): 386-91.

[13] Arai T, Numata K, Tanaka K. Ocular arterial flow hemodynamics in patients with diabetes mellitus. J Ultrasound Med. 1998; 17: 675—81.

[14] Ghanchi FD, Williamson TH, Lim CS, *et al.* Color Doppler imaging in giant cell(temporal) arteritis: serial examination and comparison with non-arteritic anterior ischaemic optic neuropathy. Eye(Lond). 1996; 10: 459-64.

[15] Goebel W, Lieb WE, Ho A, *et al.* Color Doppler imaging: a new technique to assess orbital blood flow in patients with diabetic retinopathy. Invest Ophthalmol Vis Sci. 1995; 36: 864-70.

[16] Kičová N, Bertelmann T, Irle S, *et al.* Evaluation of a posterior vitreous detachment: a comparison of biomicroscopy, B-scan echography and optical coherence tomography to surgical findings with chromodissection. Acta Ophthalmol. 2012; 90(4): 264-8.

[17] Genovesi-Ebert F, Rizzo S, Chiellini S, *et al.* Reliability of standardized echography before vitreoretinal surgery for proliferative diabetic retinopathy. Ophthalmologica. 1998; 212 Suppl 1: 91-2.

[18] Trible JR, Anderson DR. Factors associated with retrobulbar hemodynamic measurements at variable intraocular pressure. J Glaucoma. 1998; 7: 33-8.

[19] Rankin SJ. Color-Doppler imaging of the retrobulbar circulation in glaucoma. Surv Ophthalmol. 1999; 43 Suppl 1: S176-82.

CHAPTER 7

Ultrasound and Ocular Trauma

Pedro Romero-Aroca[1,*], Manuel Montero-Jaime[2,*] and Demetrio A Ramos-Dominguez[3]

[1]Department of Ophthalmology, [2]Department of Radiology University Hospital Sant Joan, Rovira & Virgili University, Pere Virgili Health Research Institute, IISPV, Reus, Spain and [3]Department of Ophthalmology, Hospital Star Médica, Instituto de Seguridad y Servicios Sociales de los Trabajadores del Estado, ISSSTE, Mérida, Mexico

Abstract: The ultrasound in ocular traumatism is an essential technique of examination. It is the gold standard technique in case of intraocular foreign body. In these patients magnetic resonance is completely avoided, in a possible metallic foreign body. The ocular trauma makes difficult the posterior segment visualization and echography helps us determine retina lesions, as retinal detachment. The echography is essential for determining intraocular foreign body location.

Keywords: Ocular injury, Globus rupture, penetrating ocular injuries, ocular perforation, intraocular foreign body.

INTRODUCTION

The diagnosis of ocular trauma is made, basically, by the physical examination of the anterior and posterior segment of the same [1-3]. The ocular globe is an organ prominently located on the front of the orbit and possesses a structure that could be defined as cystic due to the presence of various fluid-filled cavities in it; this organ is ideal for exploration by imaging techniques such as echography [4, 5]. The exploration by imaging techniques is important for the presence of an ocular trauma, especially to exclude the presence of intraocular foreign bodies, perforations of the ocular globe or ruptures of the same that in the simple physical examination could not be sometimes determined. Although, ocular echography gives us a lot of information for a traumatized eye, and especially with media opacity; in certain circumstances, other techniques of imaging as computed tomography [CT] can provide us more data [6-8]. Also in some cases, nuclear

***Corresponding authors Manuel Montero-Jaime:** Hospital Universitario Sant Joan, Avda. Doctor Josep Laporte 1 Reus, Spain; E-mail: mmontero@grupsagessa.com
Pedro Romero Aroca: Hospital Universitario Sant Joan, Avda. Doctor Josep Laporte 1 Reus, Spain; E-mail: pormero@grupsagessa.com

Pedro Romero-Aroca and Manuel Montero-Jaime (Eds.)

magnetic resonance [MR] is essential in exploring of the same orbit [9-11]. Ultrasound is also important in the posterior, following the treatment of trauma itself to determine the evolution of lesions, such as the presence of serous or hemorrhagic choroidal detachment (Fig. **1**), or the appearance of new lesions such as retinal detachment and retinal vitreous proliferation. Moreover, the dynamic exploration of the ocular globe, which allows the ocular ultrasound, is helpful under certain conditions as in the case of presence of vitreous hemorrhage to rule out if it is associated or not with retinal detachment.

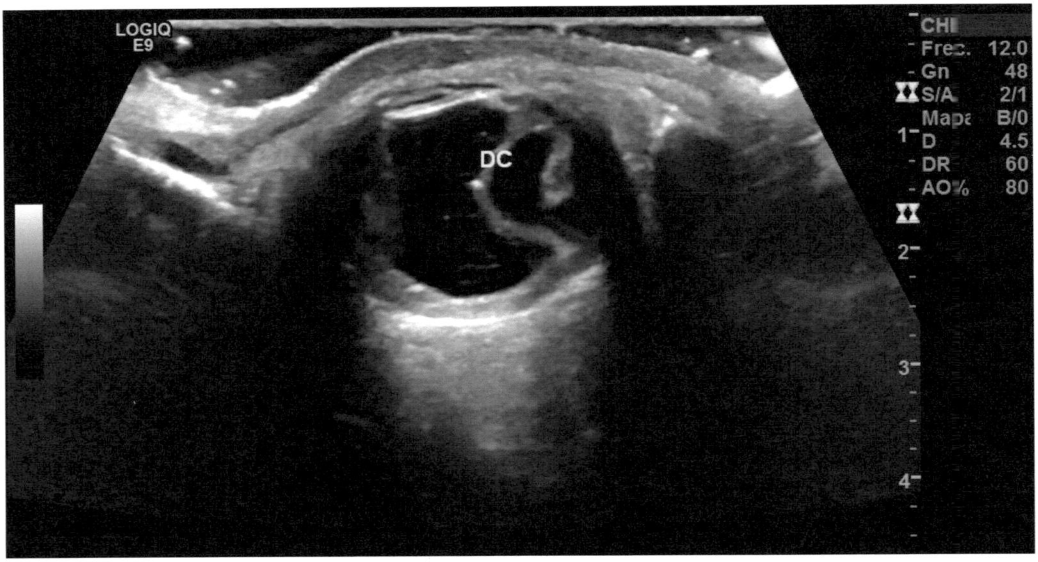

Figure 1: Choroidal detachment [DC], secondary to intraocular hypotension after vitrectomy.

CLASSIFICATION

The classification of ocular trauma is the internationally recommended [The Birmingham Eye Trauma Terminology system, BETT], which divides the trauma in [12, 13]:

- Closed ocular globe is further classified in: blunt or lamellar lacerations.
- Open ocular globe includes: rupture of the ocular globe, or penetrating wounds of the globe [an entry wound without an exit wound of the globe], or perforating injuries [double wound of the ocular globe, in and out], or presence of intraocular foreign bodies.

The diagnostic imaging techniques used and the devices currently in use at our hospital are:

- Ocular ultrasound by GE LOGIC 700 with linear probes 7 to 12 MHz
- The TC by GE HI-SPEED
- By GE1 TESLA MRI.

THE TRAUMATIC EYE

Once the ocular trauma is produced, we follow a series of steps in its evaluation. We 1 perform this through a complete medical history that includes: the location of the trauma, the description of the mechanism and circumstances of the case [for example, major trauma with footballs probably only give place to blunt trauma], the elapsed time since the moment of the trauma, and the possibility of foreign bodies in the eye as a consequence of the type of trauma that has taken place. Then, a full scan of the eye is done that includes visual acuity, visual field, anterior segment examination by slit lamp, intraocular pressure determination and fundus examination. The ocular globe exploration by imaging techniques helps to determine the ocular globe condition, the presence of derived complications from the trauma, and the presence of intraocular foreign bodies. We can use the B-type ocular ultrasound, or two-dimensional, and the computed tomography [CT] as diagnostic methods that give better information. As a secondary term, we have the magnetic resonance imaging [MRI] as a technique of secondary information with ocular trauma's cases, rather than its use in cases where the presence of metallic origin intraocular foreign bodies is suspected, because of its contraindication [9, 14-16]. In addition to this, it is important to highlight that, in many cases, the information given by the patient, or the preliminary exploration, cannot just rule out this presence; and this is a reason to exclude the use of MRI. B-Mode ocular ultrasound has the following advantages: it gives us a real picture in motion of the ocular globe and the orbit; it allows us to obtain images with good resolution of intraocular structures, by being able to observe axial and radial cuts of the ocular globe; it allows us to keep track of the trauma evolution, by being able to obtain serial images in the following days [important fact in choroidal hemorrhage or serous detachments monitoring]; and finally, the most attractive aspect of this technology is its low cost. However, ultrasound has a number of disadvantages: it requires a direct contact of the ultrasound transducer with the eye bringing a risk of extrusion of the ocular content, in the presence of perforating or penetrating wounds of the ocular globe [4, 5, 17-19]; it is not useful in case of orbit fracture; and it requires a learning technique, which is not easy at all [20].

CLOSED-GLOBE INJURIES, BRUISES

These injuries cause a wide lesions spectrum in various intraocular structures due to the antero-posterior compression of the ocular globe with the corresponding shift in the equatorial plane [21-23].

LESIONS AT THE ANTERIOR CHAMBER LEVEL

1. Hyphema and Lesions at the Iris Level

At the level of the anterior chamber, we can observe the detachment of the iris and the display of blood in the anterior chamber, or hyphema, with the increase of intraocular pressure secondary; in this case, the ultrasound is useful in the determination of this detachment, especially if we use frequencies of 18 MHz [24, 25]. The presence of hyphema, previously described, can be seen on B-mode ultrasound, and we also see its displacement with the eye and head movements, which we can see in acute hyphemas, but those hyphemas with long time evolution we observe that the hyphema remains stable and does not move with the eye movements. In addition, these injuries can lead to a dislocation of the lens, not only in the anterior chamber, but also in the vitreous cavity; the ultrasound is useful to determine the lens condition inside the eye, because after a trauma of this magnitude, it tends to be accompanied of hemorrhage in the anterior chamber [hyphema] and/or vitreous cavity making the vision of the lens difficult. Also in cataract surgery patients, we can observe the condition of the intraocular lens [IOL] inside the vitreous, with the presence of subluxation, or dislocation, of the IOL inside the vitreous being common.

LESIONS IN THE VITREOUS CAVITY LEVEL

1. Vitreous Hemorrhage

The presence of vitreous hemorrhage in blunt trauma forces us to perform an ultrasound as a first choice; its purpose is intended to determine the presence of retinal detachment and the ocular globe's perforation or penetration. Ultrasound is very sensitive in determining the presence of vitreous hemorrhage, by increasing its echogenicity as days pass by; and if it has been caused for penetration of a foreign body, the entry route may clearly be observed (Fig. **2**). In case of the presence of vitreous hemorrhage, the monitoring of the same with ultrasound is excellent because it determines its reabsorption and the possible occurrence of complications as retinal detachment. A new ultrasound should be performed every 4 months until its complete reabsorption. In ultrasound, the vitreous hemorrhage is identified as the echogenic material that moves freely in the vitreous chamber along the eye movements. The evolution can lead to reabsorption, or to the organization, with the formation of fibrovascular vitreous scars that induces a retinal detachment. This evolution is more common in massive bleeding, so that serial studies are essential. As for it, the CT shows a high density mass barely defined. Regarding to the ultrasound, it does not define the scarring vitreous disorders.

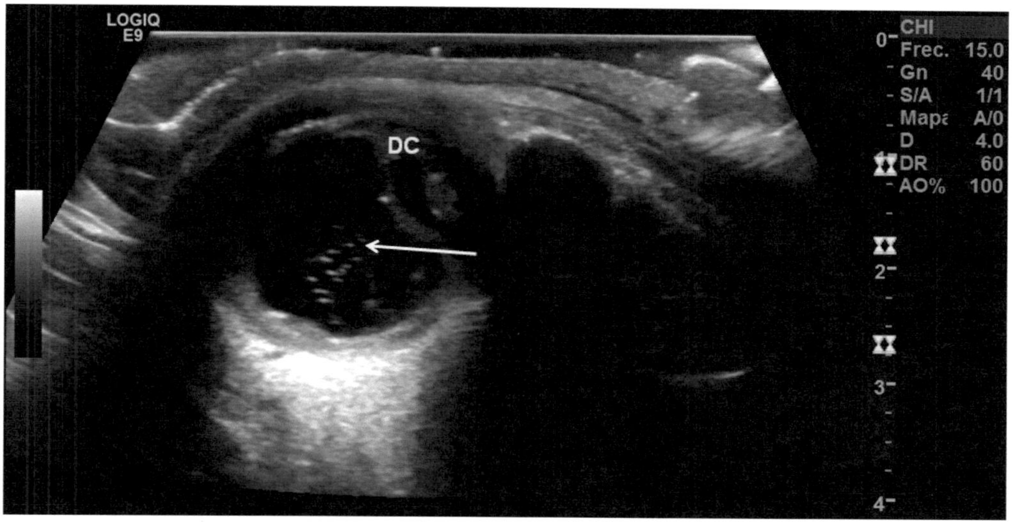

Figure 2: Vitreous tract due intraocular foreign body [arrow indicates multiples foreign bodies into the vitreous], DC = choroid detachment.

2. Retinal Detachment

One of the complications of the blunt traumas is the occurrence of retinal detachment that is observe on the ultrasound as a linear separation of the retina remaining attached at some point near the papilla (Fig. **3**). In case of complete detachment, we observe the typical V-shape image in the papilla (Fig. **4**) as starting point like a zone of maximum grip. The toughest thing to observe is the occurrence of tears in the retinal periphery; in the blunt traumas, it has been estimated that in a 25% there was an avulsion of the vitreous base, and therefore, risk of tearing; in the ultrasound, we see it as a hyper reflective small area attached to the peripheral retina that is not modified along the eye movement. It considers differential diagnosis with bands of peripheral vitreous scarring, generally with poor movement.

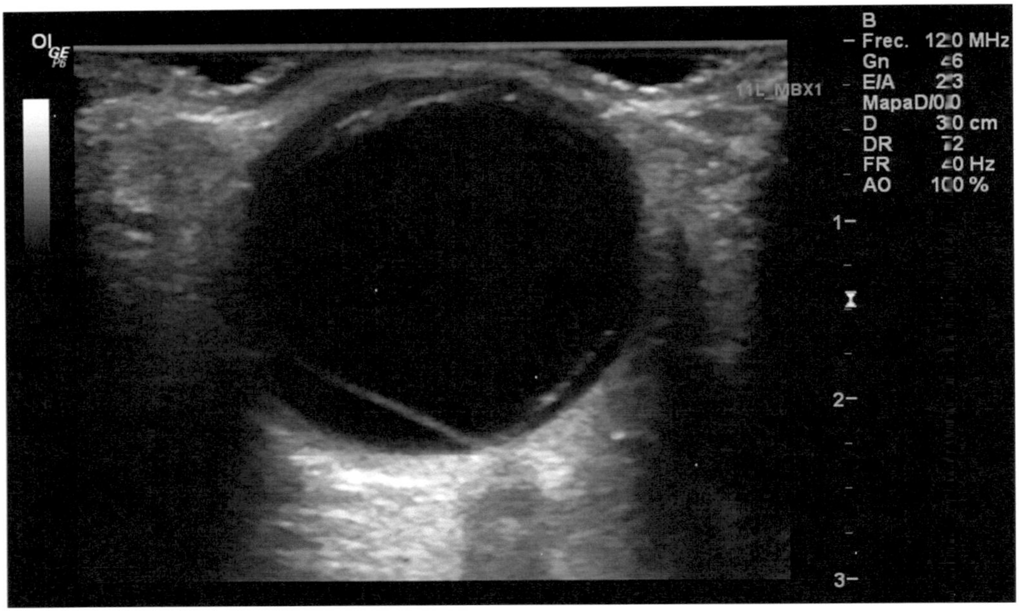

Figure 3: Retinal detachment, attached to optical nerve.

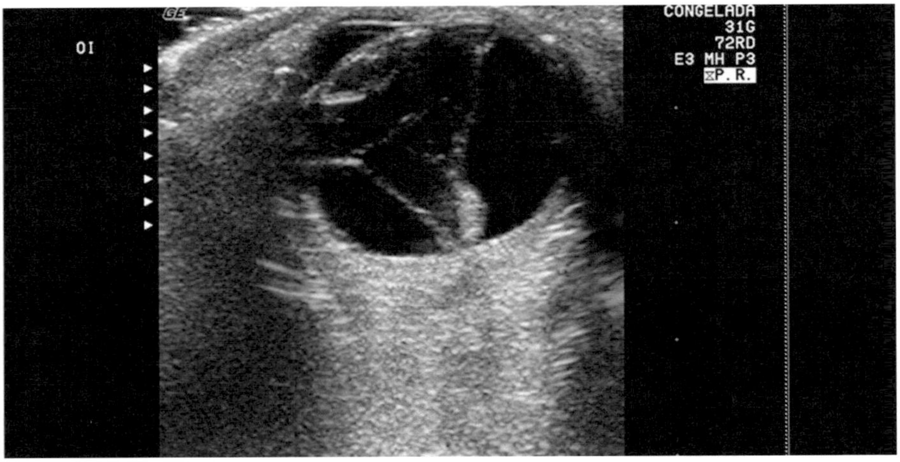

Figure 4: Chronic retinal detachment, a tunnel Y shaped is formed by a rigid detached retina.

3. Proliferative Vitreo-Retinopathy [PVR]

In the evolution of blunt traumas, proliferative vitreo-retinopathies [PVR] secondary or not to a companion retinal detachment may eventually succeed; in this case, the echography signs are defined by the existence of thick lines with retinal attachment, barely modified by the eye movements, and with occasionally demonstrable neovascularization in Color-Doppler ultrasound [26].

4. Traumatic Choroidal Abnormalities

In blunt traumas, alterations in the choroid level may also be observed, visible on ultrasound as serous or choroidal hemorrhage, but these are more common in cases of open-globe. Finally, albeit rare, there may appear an avulsion of the optic nerve, which is demonstrated by the use of CT mainly [27, 28].

OCULAR OPEN-GLOBE INJURIES

The open-globe injuries can be wall perforations; the perforating wounds generally occur parallel to the corneal limbus at the level of the sclera. In this case, we see in the ultrasound a discontinuity at the level of the sclera; this discontinuity can be observed with greater accuracy in the CT. The presence of an entry and an exit wound is called ocular perforation; this is similar to the previous case, and we are able to see in both the ultrasound and the CT (Fig. **5**), a discontinuity of the scleral wall.

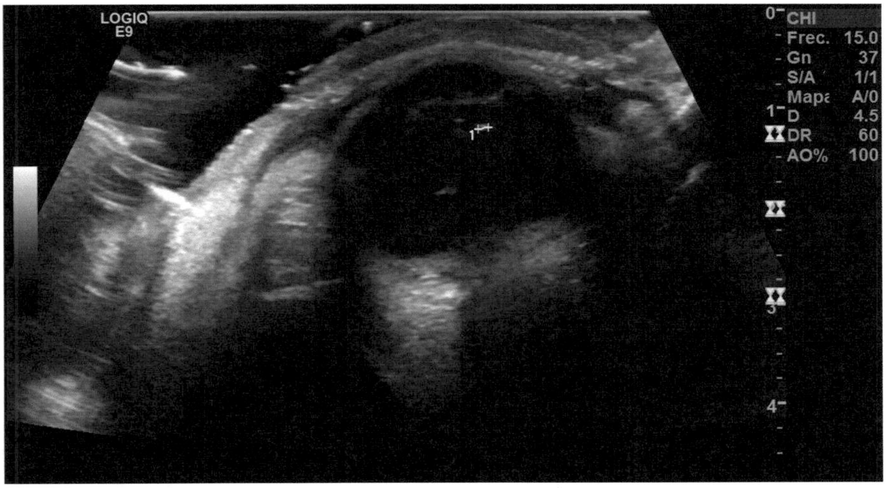

Figure 5: Posterior globe rupture seen in echography, the antero-posterior axis has been decreased, and the posterior sclera concavity has disappeared.

In both cases mentioned before, there are a series of injuries that often accompany them, such as: the vitreous hemorrhage previously described or the presence of lesions in the choroid in accord, basically, with the detachment of the same.

- Full: Convex lines projecting from the anterior pole to the posterior pole of the eye. The posterior aspect is not anchored in the optical disc. In cases of bleeding, the suprachoroidal space appears filled with echogenic material in the ultrasound and hyper-dense in the CT.

- Partial: A convex thick line is identified in the nasal, temporal or both sides. Externally, we appreciate echogenic material or high-dense according to the imaging technique used in the cases of bleeding.

- Serous: This occurs due to the accumulation of non-bloody fluid: in the ultrasound, it is identified by its low echogenicity; and in the CT, it is identified by its low density. It is often associated to surgery and penetrating trauma. It is also associated to penetrating trauma, the hemorrhagic one, as well as the eye contusion.

The hemorrhagic choroidal detachment has a worse prognosis than the serous one. The ultrasound is useful to determine its evolution; and with the passage of days, we observe a central liquefaction at the level of the choroid with a progressive decrease of the echogenicity that allows, within 10-14 days, performing a surgical drain of it [29, 30]. As vitreous incarceration in the wound may occur in cases of ocular globe's perforation or penetration, we could see as a hypoechoic area attached to the wound and partially mobilized from it. This type of injuries lead, much more often, to the emergence of PVR, which pulls the retina from the vitreous, making visible the presence of a tractional retinal detachment; in this case, we observe in ultrasound the presence of the triangle sign in contrast to the tractional or rhegmatogenous detachment. Finally, the open-globe injuries may be accompanied with the presence of an intraocular foreign body. In this case, if the foreign body is metallic [31], the CT is more useful than ultrasound because it allows to determine its position inside the ocular globe (Figs. **6**, 7); but if the foreign body is non-metallic, the ultrasound is superior in this case. In case of a non-metallic foreign body, the ultrasound allows us to identify the position of the foreign body inside the ocular globe, especially through the use of kinetic ultrasound that gives us an approximated idea of its location inside the vitreous cavity, which is adjacent to the eye layers [retina-choroid] or inside of them. Also, it can give us information about the route followed through the ocular globe at the moment of the penetration, sometimes as a trickle of foreign body debris located through the vitreous. Also in extra ocular foreign body in contact with the eye from orbit, we can observe the presence of eye damage to the area surrounding the foreign body.

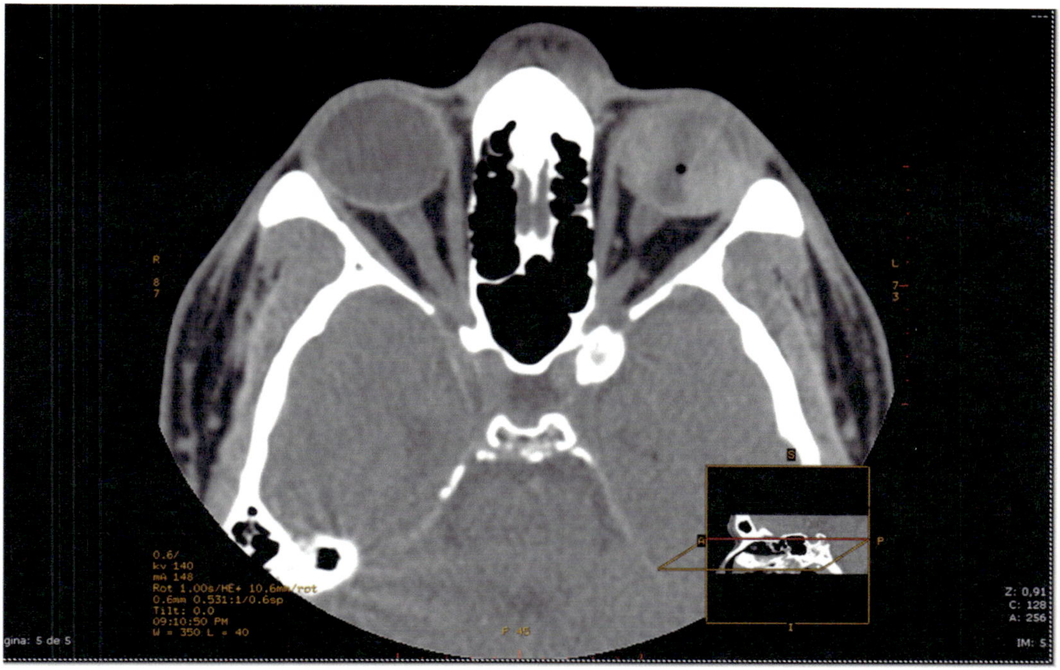

Figure 6: Nonmetallic foreign body seen in computed tomography (CT).

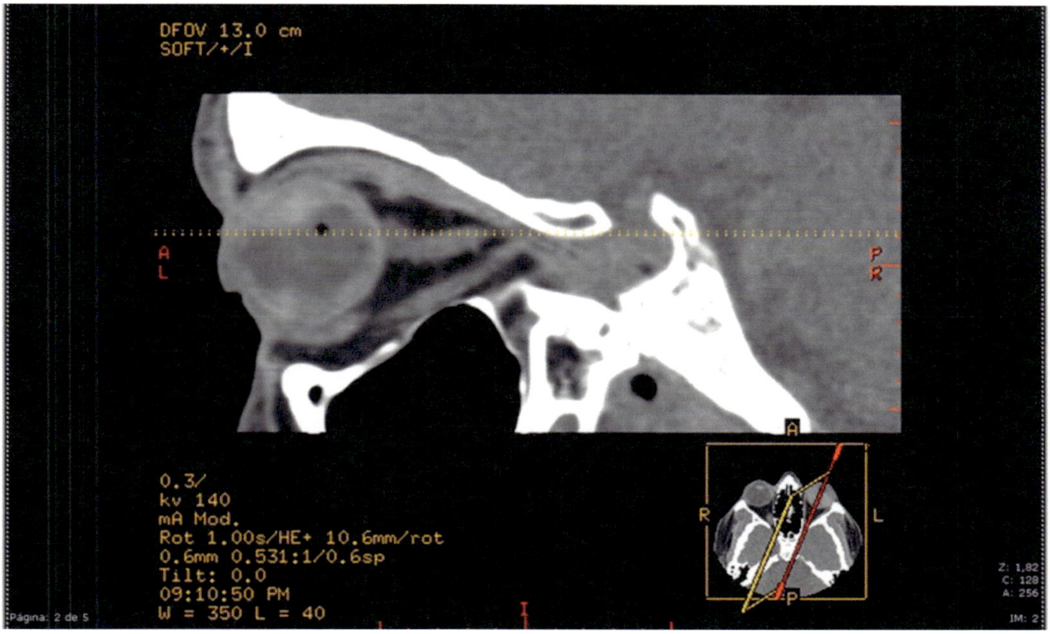

Figure 7: Nonmetallic foreign body seen in computed tomography (CT).

CONCLUDING REMARKS

Echography is basic in ocular trauma examination. Most of the ocular injuries include intraocular perforation or penetration according to the international classification. In these cases, the presence of palpebral closure with difficulty in globe examination, indicates the ultrasound examination. Even in intraocular body suspicions, other techniques as magnetic resonance are avoided, and only the echography permits to detect the foreign body location.

ACKNOWLEDGEMENTS

Declared None.

CONFLICT OF INTEREST

The authors confirm that this chapter contents have no conflict of interest.

REFERENCES

[1] Wagner PJ, Lang GK Mechanical ocular trauma. Curr Opin Ophthalmol. 1996; 7: 57-64.
[2] Harlan JB Jr, Pieramici DJ. Evaluation of patients with ocular trauma. Ophthalmol Clin North Am. 2002; 15: 153-61.
[3] Kubal WS. The pathological globe: clinical and imaging analysis. Semin Ultrasound CT MR. 1997; 18: 423-36.
[4] Fielding JA. The assessment of ocular injury by ultrasound. Clin Radiol. 2004; 59: 301-12.
[5] Ozdal MP, Mansour M, Deschenes J. Ultrasound biomicroscopic evaluation of the traumatized eyes. Eye. 2003; 17: 467-72.
[6] Joseph DP, Pieramici DJ, Beauchamp NJ Jr. Computed tomography in the diagnosis and prognosis of open-globe injuries. Ophthalmology. 2000; 107: 1899-906.
[7] Artmann H, Grau H, Losche CC. The significance of computed tomography in ophthalmologic diagnosis. I: The place of computed tomography, indications, study technics, anatomic representation, computed tomography of ocular globe and orbital injuries. Radiol Diagn(Berl). 1989; 30: 621-8.
[8] Ho VH, Wilson MW, Fleming JC, *et al.* Retained intraorbital metallic foreign bodies. Ophthal Plast Reconstr Surg. 2004; 20: 232-6.
[9] Lustrin ES, Brown JH, Novelline R, *et al.* Radiologic assessment of trauma and foreign bodies of the eye and orbit. Neuroimaging Clin N Am. 1996; 6: 219-37.
[10] Bair RL, Wells RG, Massaro BM, *et al.* Imaging in orbital trauma. Semin Ophthalmol. 1994; 9: 185-92.
[11] Nelson CC, Cartwright MJ. Orbital diagnosis and imaging. Curr Opin Ophthalmol. 1992; 3(5): 623-31.
[12] Kuhn F, Morris R, Witherspoon CD, *et al.* A standardized classification of ocular trauma. Ophthalmology. 1996; 103: 240-3.
[13] Kuhn F, Morris R, Witherspoon CD, *et al.* The Birmingham Eye Trauma Terminology system(BETT). J Fr Ophtalmol. 2004; 27: 206-10.
[14] Fulcher TP, Mc Nab AA, Sullivan TJ. Clinical features and management of intraorbital foreign bodies. Ophthalmology. 2002; 109: 494-500.
[15] Michon J, Liu D. Intraorbital foreign bodies. Semin Ophthalmol. 1994; 9: 193-9.
[16] Ta CN, Bowman RW. Hyphema caused by a metallic intraocular foreign body during magnetic resonance imaging. Am J Ophthalmol. 2000; 129: 533-4.

[17] Fielding JA. Ocular ultrasound. Clin Radiol. 1996; 51: 533-44.
[18] Fielding JA. Imaging the eye with ultrasound.Br J Hosp Med. 1992; 47: 805-15.
[19] Mittra RA, Mieler WF. Controversies in the management of open-globe injuries involving the posterior segment. Surv Ophthalmol. 1999; 44: 215-25.
[20] Bair RL, Wells RG, Massaro BM, *et al.* Imaging in orbital trauma. Semin Ophthalmol. 1994; 9: 185-92.
[21] Turbin RE, Maxwell DN, Langer PD, *et al.* Patterns of transorbital intracranial injury: a review and comparison of occult and non-occult cases. Surv Ophthalmol. 2006; 51: 449-60.
[22] Bilyk JR, Joseph MP. Traumatic optic neuropathy. Semin Ophthalmol. 1994; 9: 200-11.
[23] Steinsapir KD, Goldberg RA. Traumatic optic neuropathy. Surv Ophthalmol. 1994; 38: 487-518.
[24] Ishikawa H, Schuman JS. Related Articles, Anterior segment imaging: ultrasound biomicroscopy. Ophthalmol Clin North Am. 2004; 17: 7-20.
[25] Wolffsohn JS, Davies LN. Advances in anterior segment imaging. Curr Opin Ophthalmol. 2007; 18: 32-8.
[26] Lieb WE. Color-Doppler imaging of the eye and orbit. Radiol Clin North Am. 1998; 36: 1059-71.
[27] Foster BS, March GA, Lucarelli MJ, *et al.* Optic nerve avulsion. Arch Ophthalmol. 1997; 115: 623-30. Erratum in: Arch Ophthalmol 1997; 115: 1070.
[28] Roberts SP, Schaumberg DA, Thompson P. Traumatic avulsion of the optic nerve.Optom Vis Sci. 1992; 69: 721-7.
[29] Chu TG, Cano MR, Green RL. Massive suprachoroidal hemorrhage with central retinal apposition: A clinical and echographic study. Arch Ophthalmol 1991; 109: 1575-81.
[30] Chu TG, Green RL. Suprachoroidal hemorrhage. Surv Ophthalmology 1999; 43: 471-86.
[31] Mester V, Kuhn F. Ferrous intraocular foreign bodies retained in the posterior segment: management options and results. Int Ophthalmol. 1998; 22: 355-62.

Chapter 8: Ultrasound and Eye Surgery

CHAPTER 8

Ultrasound and Eye Surgery

Pedro Romero-Aroca[1,*], Manuel Montero-Jaime[2,*], Nuria Soler[1] and Jose A Buil-Calvo[3]

[1]Department of Ophthalmology, Department of Radiology [2], University Hospital Sant Joan, Rovira & Virgili University, Pere Virgili Health Research Institute, IISPV, Reus, Spain and [3]Department of Ophthalmology, Hospital Santa Creu i Sant Pau, Universidad Autonoma de Barcelona, Barcelona, Spain

Abstract: The ultrasound in ophthalmic surgery is essential in the preoperatory stage, when media opacities cause hindrance in the retina examination. When a patient is admitted for intraocular surgery, echography is mandatory to detect possible intraocular diseases as retinal detachment. In postoperative status, the patients need echographies if new media opacities appear as in case of postoperative hemorrhages in a vitrectomy surgery. In these cases the echography visualizes the posterior pole and permits to establish a correct diagnosis and a postoperative therapy.

Keywords: Cataract, lens luxation, intraocular lens luxation, retinal detachment, vitrectomy, periphery new vessels, tractional retinal detachment, vitreous hemorrhage, choroidal hemorrhage, malignant glaucoma.

INTRODUCTION

In this chapter, we describe the ultrasound utility in preoperative and postoperative diagnosis of different ocular entities prone to surgery and divide the different ocular pathologies according to the ocular segment affected. Many of the entities described in this chapter have already been described in previous chapters; therefore the following descriptions are short, and they refer to their corresponding chapters. A different matter is the case of the disease affecting the anterior segment, especially the lens; since this is the subject that we insist with most attention in this chapter, by describing the various pathologies affecting the anterior segment and its control using ultrasound.

ULTRASOUND IN CATARACT SURGERY

Cataract is, by far, the most common cause of ocular media opacification; thus, it

***Corresponding author Pedro Romero Aroca:** Hospital Universitario Sant Joan, Avda. Doctor Josep Laporte 1 Reus, Spain; E-mail: pormero@grupsagessa.com
Manuel Montero-Jaime: Hospital Universitario Sant Joan, Avda. Doctor Josep Laporte 1 Reus, Spain; E-mail: mmontero@grupsagessa.com

is the first reason that led us to call for ultrasound for the posterior segment exploration, since all the methods we currently possess, as biomicroscopy fundus and optical coherence tomography [OCT], require the media to be transparent. On the other hand, the posterior segment exploration is basic and necessary in the presence of any disease affecting the lens that deserves surgery, such as cataract. Let us not forget that cataract surgery is, by far, the most frequent within ophthalmology, and it affects an important segment of the population by this type of lens opacification.

Table 1: Prevalence of cataracts in the population

Population in ages	**Prevalence of cataracts**			
	Blue Mounatain [1] Australia	**Beaver Dam [2] US**	**Framingham[3]**	**VIP [4] Australia**
49-54	2,7	1,6	No data	2,6
55-64	5,0	7,2	3,4	6,7
65-74	21,6	20,0	13,2	23,2
75-84	53,6	43,4	40,8	46,1
>85	71,7	No data	No data	61,1

In Table **1**, we see the prevalence of cataracts in the population according to various studies. As has been described, the involvement of the population served with cataracts is important, and we have to emphasize in the fact that the aging of the population leads to more patients with cataracts in the coming years, especially in western countries and even so in some of the so-called emerging markets. Besides the need for a good vision, even in advanced ages. Therefore lens surgery needs will increase, since in many cases the fundus visualization is impeded by the clouded lens. Its exploration is of great importance as ultrasound technique, and should be known to all the ophthalmologists and radiologists. The question to be addressed is when is the ultrasound scan fundus required? As it is known, we need the view of the retina to be clear in order to explore it by techniques such as fundus biomicroscopy, retinography, ophthalmoscopy or OCT. Thus, as long as the opacification of the lens affects the visualization, we can use ultrasound to explore the ocular globe.

ULTRASOUND IN CATARACT SURGERY PREOPERATIVE

1. Mature Cataract, White Cataract, Non-Fundus Visualization

The most used classification of the clouding lens is the Lens Opacities Classification System III [LOCS III], which sub classifies the opacities according to the cortex affectation [C1 to C5], the nucleus affectation [NC1 to NC5], or the posterior or anterior subcapsular affectation [P1 to P5]. The classification is graded into 5 stages from lower to higher layer opacity of the lens involved; from stage 4 opacification, it is considerably hard to view the fundus [5]; therefore, the ultrasound is of great assistance in this type of cataract, regardless of whether the fundus is seen with some difficulty, but it is still visible. In the ultrasound scan, the lens shows multiple intralenticular echoes; the appearance of these echoes is due both the presence of aqueous areas inside the lens and to the malfunction of the crystalline fibres. Special cases of opacification the white cataract, which is common in young people and in cases of blunt trauma or not; and also the hypermature cataract, which has a great nucleus and cortex opacification; or even so the ones called Morgagnian cataracts (Fig. **1**), in which the nucleus is dislocated inside the clouded lens with a cortex looking white and liquefied. In these cases, the number of echoes is much higher, and we can even see the hyper reflective nucleus inside the cavity of the lens.

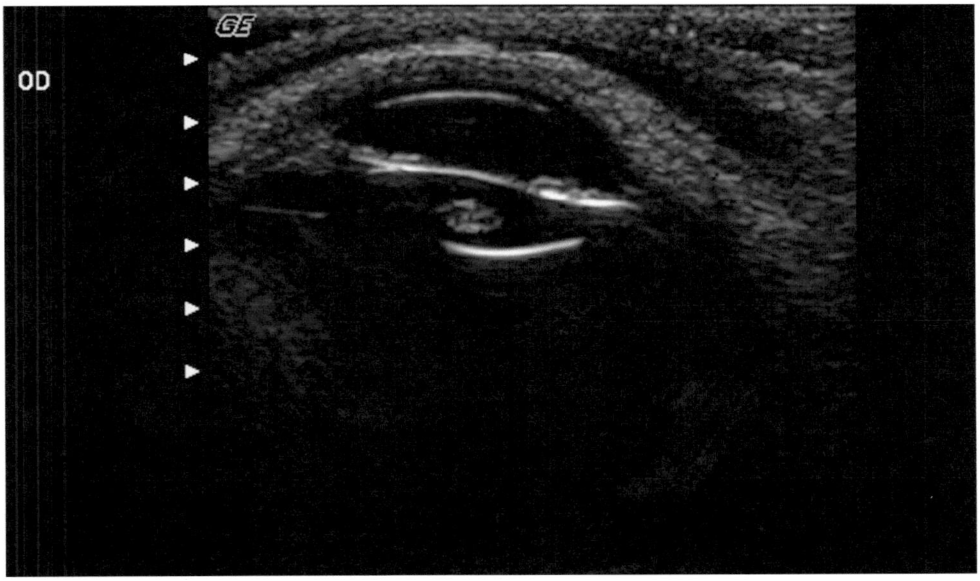

Figure 1: Nuclear cataract.

The importance of preoperative ultrasound lies on:

- Determining the axis of the eye.
- Determining, using biometrics, the calculation of power of the intraocular lens to implant.

- Disregarding the presence of other diseases at the level of the vitreous cavity or retina that would affect the outcome of the surgery.

The description of the axis measurement of the eye and the identification of the lens implant trough biometrics has been described in other chapters; we will therefore only describe the importance of ultrasound to dismiss other associated pathologies. Ultrasound allows us to systematically explore the vitreous cavity and the eye layers in search of the associated pathology, such as a retinal detachment that has not been previously detected, the presence of a vitreous hemorrhage, or conditions affecting the ocular layers as tumors. More difficult is the detection of the disease afflicting the macula and the presence of age-related macular degeneration [AMD]; stratum affected by cataracts is also common in this population. Nevertheless, we can resort to combine probes of 10 MHz for the globe exploration as a whole and to determine the presence of vitreous hemorrhage or retinal detachment using macular exploration of the area with higher frequency probes such as 20 MHz that can help us to diagnose the presence of macular holes or edema in the macular area [6, 7], if there is any AMD. If this has the exudative form, the use of Color-Doppler ultrasound can determine the existence of vascularization at the macular level. It would be identical in the case of the existence of proliferative retinopathy of any origin, as diabetes, by affecting the posterior area of the ocular globe, particularly the papilla and the vascular arcades.

LENS SUBLUXATION

One problem that can be found in cataract surgery is the intraocular lens subluxation; although, there are signs of visualization of this using anterior segment biomicroscopy; in this case, by observing the lens position, the anterior chamber depth [this being irregular in case of subluxation according to the explored axis], and the phacodonesis phenomenon [movement of the lens about its location to move the eye], the ultrasound scan can indicate us the existence of subluxation of the intraocular lens (Fig. **2**). We have to say that the most common causes, by far, are the prior eye injury and the presence of a pseudoexfoliation syndrome. The ultrasound scan should preferably be done by probes of 10 or 20 MHz; also it can be done with probes of 50 MHz [UBM] because these allow us to study in great detail the anterior segment structures, but the probes aforementioned provide enough information to know the lens condition and its position inside the anterior segment. Scanning should be done without pushing excessively on the ocular globe because it will deform the anterior segment, and it could give us a false image of the lens. Scanning is firstly performed in two axes:

one vertical to the ocular globe and the other one horizontal to the same, both perpendiculars to each other; these two images often provide us sufficient information regarding the status of the lens, but further exploration may be performed considering the time axes starting from 12 hours [or vertical] to 3 hours [or horizontal] through the 1 and 2 hours. We must determine the lens position according to the iris posterior plane and assess whether it is displaced or not; in turn, we must observe the anterior chamber depth in all areas explored.

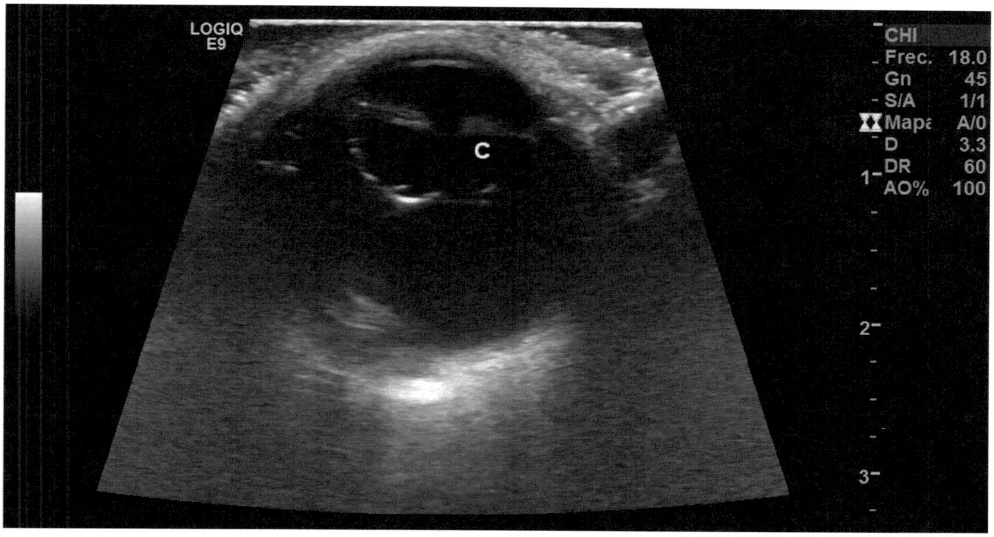

Figure 2: Intraocular lens [IOL] luxation.

LENS [CATARACT] LUXATION

In this case, the ultrasound can help us determine the presence of the lens in the vitreous cavity, and if still it is in certain extent attached, or not, to the ciliary body through the zonules. In case of lens dislocation, it is common that its cause is traumatic, so there is an associated vitreous hemorrhage that makes difficult the visualization of the fundus (Fig. **3**). It is therefore necessary to use ultrasound not only to determine the position of the dislocated lens, but also if there is associated posterior segment disease, such as retinal detachment, which would modify the approach to surgical treatment of the patient.

ULTRASOUND IN POSTOPERATIVE CATARACT SURGERY

In the cataract postoperative, the ultrasound can help us determine if the intraocular lens [IOL] implant is correctly or not in place. The probes that we use should be those previously described, 10, 20 or 50 MHz; the higher the ultrasound frequency, the higher the image resolution obtained and the IOL position inside the eye; but we must keep in mind that those structures, located more than 5 or 6 mm from the cornea, will be difficult to observe with probes greater than 20 MHz like in the case of the IOL posterior side. Therefore, with the probe of 50 MHz, we have the information of the IOL anterior side and its position in relation to the iris plane, but not all the IOL itself, especially if this is displaced into the vitreous cavity. The IOL is preferably implanted inside the capsular bag; hence the given image is of an echo behind the convex shape iris plane and is placed on the eye center, with the haptic positioned close to the ciliary body. With the ultrasound, we can see if there is an IOL tilt in relation to the iris plane, or if the haptics are outside of the ciliary body plane. In both situations we would be in an IOL subluxation. Some intraocular lenses have a lens angulation in relation to the haptics, and it is designed for a better placement inside the capsular bag. In these cases, the ultrasound is useful to us to see if the lens is properly placed in the capsular bag, or whether if the IOL is reversed by placing it. Finally, in cases of IOL dislocation inside the eye vitreous, we can determine their position inside of it by using ultrasound, and if it is accompanied by other associated pathology, such as cortical masses remains, retinal detachment and so on.

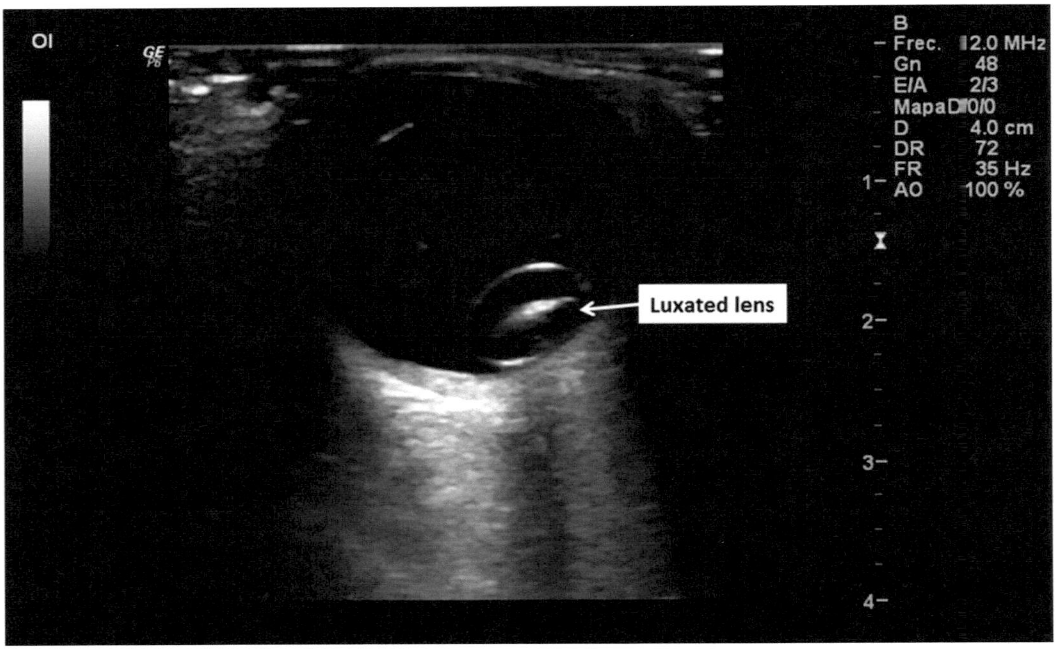

Figure 3: Lens luxation.

CHOROIDAL HEMORRHAGE, CHOROIDAL SEROUS DETACHMENT

In cases of complicated cataract surgery, it is easy to find disorders at the choroid level in the postoperative, like the case of the choroidal serous detachment, or the suprachoroidal hemorrhage. The choroidal serous detachment is associated to patients with special characteristics in their eyes, such as nanophthalmic eyes or with high hyperopia, and there also occurs serous detachment in case of filtering corneal incisions with associated hypotension; in all of them, we observe, in the ultrasound, the presence of an hypo-echogenic choroidal lifting and regular that sometimes implies the same ciliary body being, in some cases, precisely only the ciliary body which detaches. In these patients, the ultrasound allows a proper diagnosis of this disease and, in turn, its proper following. With the use of ultrasound scans in the weeks after surgery, we assess if the process is solved, or otherwise it remains stable and requires a second surgery to resolve the choroidal serous detachment. The suprachoroidal hemorrhage is a secondary hemorrhagic process of cataract surgery, and it is often complicated with a posterior capsule rupture and intraoperative episodes of hypotension. This leads to the rupture of the long posterior ciliary arteries that run through the suprachoroidal space, just below the sclera. Various systemic entities are associated with its onset such as hypertension, the use of anticoagulants, the advanced age with associated atherosclerosis, and the presence of intraoperative tachycardia crisis. In this entity, previously described in other chapters, we can observe the presence of a convex lifting at the choroidal level that protrudes into the vitreous cavity; its internal structure is hyper-echogenic and uniform; and with the passage of time, hyper-echogenic spaces occur in its interior allowing the ultrasound to follow these patients and determine if the hemorrhage is properly absorbed, or if it requires a second surgery that allows the removal of the liquefied blood through the sclera [8, 9].

MALIGNANT GLAUCOMA

The emergence of chronic glaucoma secondary to cataract surgery is usually caused by: the existence of a chronic open-angle glaucoma prior to surgery [as the most common], swelling at the camerular angle level [trabeculitis] and deposits in the same, anterior synechiae between cornea and iris at the angular level [especially in the case of extracapsular extraction], or after the use of topical steroids in the postoperative. A pupillary block glaucoma may also occur if the IOL is trapped at the pupillary level, either by its bad positioning or after an eye injury that moves forward, but now with the use of the phacoemulsification and the new foldable IOLs, this form of pupillary block glaucoma occurs more sporadically. There is also a form of glaucoma called malignant that occurs by the rotation of the ciliary body; in this way, the aqueous humor is directed toward the posterior side of the vitreous cavity rather than the anterior chamber. Besides, it is also characteristic of this form that the practice of a peripheral iridectomy, or iridotomy, does not produce any improvement and does not restore the flow of aqueous humor into the anterior chamber. The recommended treatment for these cases is extensive vitrectomy, especially by dealing with the retreat of the most anterior vitreous in touch with the iridal plane and along with the anterior hyaloid. The ultrasound helps to diagnose the two latter forms of glaucoma; in both cases, the anterior chamber is reduced with scarce aqueous humor, and we are able to observe the presence of the IOL trapped at the pupillary level in the case of pupillary block glaucoma. By contrast in the case of malignant glaucoma, the use of ultrasound between 10 and 20 MHz informs of the existence of a liquid posterior vitreous being this more compact and hyper reflective in the ultrasound [10]. The vitreous is trapped in the anterior vitreous cavity with limited movement; it is also possible to observe the rotation of the ciliary body in posterior direction, the cause of malignant glaucoma.

ANTERIOR SEGMENT SURGERY, EXCEPT FOR THE LENS

It is advisable to use immersion probes for the study of structures in the anterior segment such as the cornea, the iris, and/or the camerular angle; by using a viscoelastic substance [such as hydroxyl methylcellulose 2%] with a capsule that keeps, in turn, the eyelids separated. The probe is immersed in the viscoelastic substance, and it is directed perpendicularly to the lesion to study. It is advisable to use probes of 20 to 50 MHz [or BMU probe].

The advantages of using probes of 20 MHz include:

- Simplicity in its performance
- Ability to visualize the anterior segment with a good resolution
- Ability to analyze lesions in the ciliary body [tumors for example], since this is placed at more than 5 mm of the probe.

The advantages of using probes of 50 MHz include:

- The almost microscopic resolution of the images obtained, by allowing the visualization of thin structures as the scleral spur, and be able to separate two structures of similar reflectivity as is the case of the tumor wall of an adjacent sclera.

1. Corneal Surgery

In corneal surgery, the most common surgery in these cases is the keratoplasty for corneal opacities; the application of ultrasound can only provide us preoperative information about the condition of the lens, of the vitreous cavity, and of the posterior wall of the eye, if there is any corneal opacity that hinders the view of the posterior pole. As a general rule, if the complications following surgery that affect the anterior segment are visible, it does not require ultrasound; and in case of occurrence of a pupillary block glaucoma or a malignant glaucoma, the application of ultrasound reports the ocular globe condition just as it is described in the preceding chapter.

2. Iris Surgery

The iris surgery is usually performed on tumors that appear in the same; the description of these has been made in a previous chapter. The study of these tumors benefits itself from the use of ultrasound with probes of 20 and 50 MHz. It is important to measure the two largest diameters and thickness of the tumor, to locate the tumor in relation to the pupillary margin, and to analyze the tumor echo-structure [reflectivity, attenuation and homogeneity]. As it is described in the corresponding chapter of eye injuries, the exploration of the case of eye injury with involvement of the iris is preferable to perform it with 20 MHz probes, being able to determine the existence of tears or detachments at the level of the root of the iris, as well as the presence of hyphema.

3. Glaucoma Surgery

Glaucoma is classified as:

- Chronic Glaucoma or open-angle [a subgroup would be normal-tension glaucoma] or closed-angle [by pupillary block or plateau iris syndrome]
- Acute Glaucoma or closed-angle by pupillary block or anterior segment postoperative malignant [usually cataract]
- Secondary glaucoma or Neovascular
- Congenital Glaucoma

Besides laser treatment [by means of argon laser trabeculoplasty for chronic glaucoma, and the iridotomies with the Nd-YAG laser for acute angle closure glaucoma], the glaucoma surgical treatment includes trabeculectomy surgery, and recently, the non-penetrating surgical techniques of glaucoma have been incorporated, in case of chronic glaucoma; we also have to describe the surgery with the use of valves in cases of complicated glaucoma or neovascular glaucoma.

4. Ultrasound in Postoperative Glaucoma Surgery

The ultrasound examination of glaucoma has its indication in the knowledge of the iridocorneal angle's condition that we can determine with probes of 10 and 20 MHz, but we can observe the details much better with the probe of 50 MHz; nevertheless, if there is visualization of the iridocorneal angle, the best technique for exploring is gonioscopy [11, 12]. Additionally, we may explore by means of Color-Doppler ultrasound the blood flow velocity at the level of the central retinal artery, the posterior ciliary artery, and ophthalmic artery; its usefulness has been described in the corresponding chapter in this book. The ultrasound usefulness in case of pupillary block glaucoma and malignant glaucoma secondary to anterior segment surgery has already been described in the preceding chapter. We pointed out that in case of acute pupillary block glaucoma that is not postoperative; it could be useful for us to determine by means of ultrasound the presence of associated pathology prior to surgery or iridectomy by laser surgery Nd-YAG or iridotomy.

5. Ultrasound in Postoperative Glaucoma Surgery

In postoperative glaucoma surgery, the ultrasound has its place in helping the diagnosis from possible complications; its usefulness lies mainly in the study of the complications occurred after the practice of a filtering surgery [trabeculectomy] with or without the use of drain valves.

HERNIA OF THE IRIS

The herniation of the iris through the trabeculectomy scleral flap can lead to its obstruction and failure of the surgery; generally, they are visible through the anterior segment biomicroscopy and the iridocorneal angle study, but ultrasound helps us to observe this herniation, particularly being useful with probes of 50 MHz

OCULAR HYPOTENSION

The excessive strain of aqueous humor by trabeculectomy may lead to postoperative hypotension, which is recovered after few days, but we must not forget that in case of ocular hypotension, a serous choroidal detachment and an increase in the choroidal thickness may appear (Fig. **4**), which is often ophthalmoscopically visible, but that in case of media opacity, the ultrasound will reveal it as it was described in the corresponding chapter; besides it will be useful for us in order to differentiate the choroidal detachment from a possible suprachoroidal hemorrhage, although in the latter case the intraocular pressure is usually high.

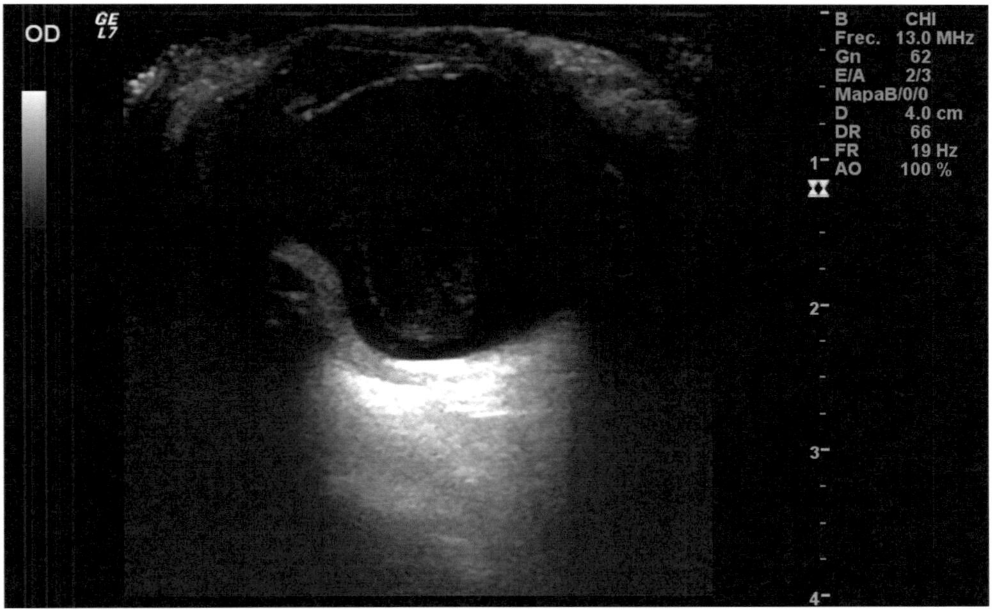

Figure 4: Increase choroidal thickness (arrow) due ocular hypotension.

POSTERIOR SEGMENT SURGERY [VITREO-RETINAL]

The ultrasound scan has a great importance, by far, in vitreo-retinal surgery, since in these cases the media are opacified with great frequency, and thus it is difficult to study the visualization problems affecting the posterior segment. Furthermore, the ultrasound will be useful for us for a postoperative control of patients in many cases, indicating a new surgical intervention in some entities occurring in the postoperative period. In Chapter 5, we have extensively described the usefulness of ultrasound in the posterior segment pathology; therefore, the mission of this chapter is not to repeat what it has already been explained, but to guide the description of the various entities affecting the surgical posterior segment, and to give a pattern of preoperative and postoperative behavior in those exclusive surgical entities affecting the posterior segment.

1. Scleral Surgery for Retinal Detachment

The scleral surgery for retinal detachment includes the closure of one or several tears by means of extrascleral cryotherapy or laser photocoagulation, and it is accompanied with scleral indentation performed by a circular silicone procedure [this is most used procedure in scleral surgeries] or either radial [with sponge-type explants]. The use of these explants is not exempted of complications after surgery, in which ultrasound can help us with a correct diagnosis.

2. Ultrasound in the Preoperative Ocular Surgery

The indications to perform an ultrasound to a retinal detachment prior surgery include:

- In suspicion of a retinal detachment existence, in case of media opacity that does not allow to visualize well the fundus of the eye in order to confirm the presence of retinal detachment.
- To dismiss an exudative retinal detachment secondary to another disease, it could be of tumoral origin, such as choroidal melanoma.
- Discard a tractional origin of the same, although, in these cases, if the media allows it, the fundus examination by biomicroscopy can give us a diagnosis.
- In cases of vitreoretinal proliferation, especially if the central tunnel is closed, and the papilla is not observed.

Using ultrasound, we can determine the shape and size of the retinal detachment; besides, it can also help us to establish a correct differential diagnosis with the exudative or tractional type forms of retinal detachment. Recently, series have been published in which the presence of peripheral retinal tears without associated retinal detachment can be observed, being useful in the ultrasound of patients with media opacities, as is the case of cataract or pseudophakic patients with significant opacity in the posterior capsule; situations like this hinder the retinal periphery visualization [13].

3. Usefulness of Ultrasound in the Normal Postoperative

The used scleral procedures are anechogenic to ultrasound, with hyper-echogenic interference in its earlier portion, which involves a posterior acoustic shadow; we are able to easily detect the scleral procedure's position in the equator's anterior area of the ocular globe, shaped as band that is indented in the sclera towards the ocular globe interior. The used sponges for radial indentation procedures are hyperechogenic, and they involve a posterior acoustic shadow and a discrete noisy device in the ultrasound; its location is more difficult in the case of not knowing its position in the eye, since the procedure is placed only in retinal tear area.

4. Ultrasound in the Complications of Scleral Surgery

Excessive compression of the scleral procedure: The first complication in the use of circular scleral procedures is the excessive compression of the same above the sclera and its layers and adjacent vessels, by leading to a difficulty in the venous return by compressing the vorticose veins; it is described that even with a compression, which can be considered normal, the scleral procedures increase the intraocular pressure.

In the most extreme case, an excessive compression will result in:

- Choroidal serous detachment
- Anterior ischemia syndrome

The ultrasound findings in choroidal serous detachment have been previously described in another chapter; it is enough to note here that we can observe a convex and regular bulging in the eye wall, which extends from the scleral spur to the vorticose veins; the union between the bulged area and the normal eye wall is made abruptly and is convex, which allows us to differentiate this situation from a retinal detachment. The content of the bulge is anechogenic as befits the accumulation of serous fluid from choroidal vessels. Anterior ischemia syndrome associates: episcleral hyperaemia, corneal edema with Descemet's folds, Tyndall effect in the aqueous humor, unreactive pupil, iris rubeosis, and high intraocular pressure in most cases; although, in some cases, the pressure may be normal or low because of ciliary body level ischemia altering the aqueous humor production. The diagnosis is mainly clinical, and the ultrasound only can help us observe the indentation extent of the scleral procedure.

5. Scleral Procedure Dislocation

In this case, the scleral procedure dislocates into a posterior direction of the ocular globe; in these cases, the ultrasound will show us the position of the scleral procedure regarding the ocular globe.

6. New Retinal Detachment

The recurrence of retinal detachment in patients who had had a scleral surgery can reach to 20% of the cases; in this situation, the ultrasound can help us see the new detachment, especially in swollen eyes after the cataract surgery and a poor mydriasis. The images obtained are typical of a retinal detachment.

7. Vitreoretinal Proliferation [VRP]

The appearance of vitreoretinal proliferation in the retinal detachment postoperative occurs after the passage of cells from the retinal pigment epithelium into the vitreous cavity, its subsequent retinal deposit, and its transformation in inflammatory cells producing fibrin that will traction the retina when it contracts. The early stages of VRP [stages A and B] are virtually invisible to the ultrasound study; only from stage C, we observe typical signs of VRP on ultrasound (Fig. **5**).

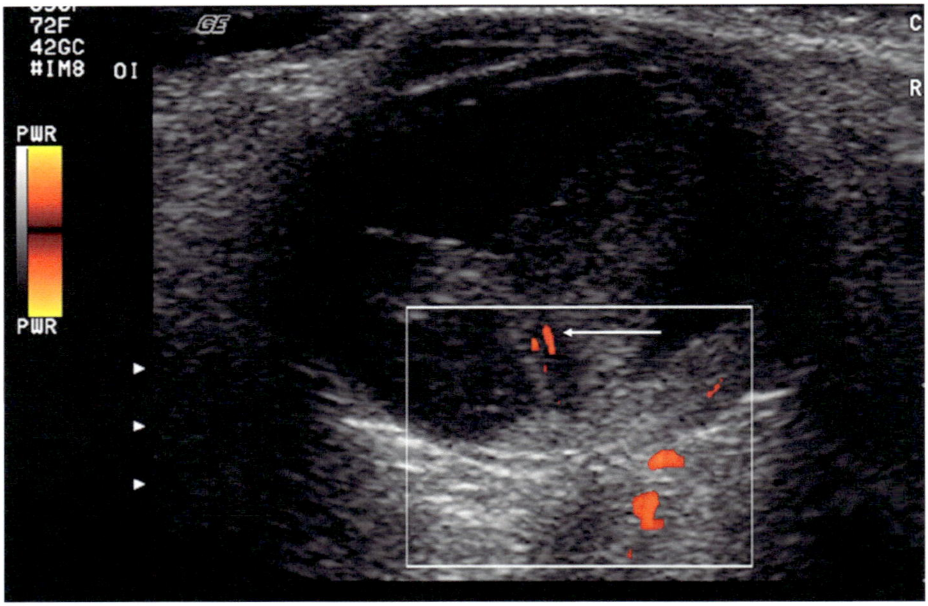

Figure 5: Proliferation vitreous-retina (PVR), tunnel shaped form, color doppler indicate the central artery between the tunnel white arrow).

- ➢ In ultrasound we are able to see:
  - o The presence of a more echogenic vitreous
  - o The appearance of echogenic pre-retinal membranes

- o Thickening of the posterior hyaloid
- o Retinal detachment that remains fixed with little movement
- o Thickening of the retina

8. Choroidal Hemorrhage

The occurrence of suprachoroidal hemorrhage after a scleral surgery for retinal detachment is not exceptional, especially if it has been associated with scleral drainage during surgery; the signs that we observe in the ultrasound have been already described above, and they include an extension of physical features similar to the serous choroidal detachment, by being bulky sometimes and with an echogenic content but not uniform heterogeneous.

POSTERIOR VITRECTOMY

The introduction of three-port pars plana vitrectomy revolutionized the treatment of vitreous and retina diseases, but at the same time, this surgery is not exempt from complications. As we have described throughout other chapters, the ultrasounds are highly useful in the diagnosis of different diseases affecting the eye socket, both to assess the prior and post situation of the surgery. Currently, posterior vitrectomy surgery includes different incision techniques; in this way, we have nowadays vitrectomies of 20, 23, and 25 gauges of incision; the latter two do not require sutures at the end of surgery. It presents a series of specific complications, mainly derived from the postoperative hypotony.

Most common indications for posterior vitrectomy:

- ➢ Retinal detachment [rhegmatogenous or tractional]
- ➢ Fibrovascular proliferation
- ➢ Vitreous hemorrhage
- ➢ Vitreous opacities [posterior uveitis]
- ➢ Macular hole
- ➢ Epiretinal membrane
- ➢ Tractional macular edema

Preoperative ultrasound examination, in case of posterior vitrectomy, includes all the conditions described in the chapter on the posterior segment ultrasound, which we refer to the reader.

ULTRASOUND IN POSTOPERATIVE VITRECTOMY

1. Anterior Fibrovascular Proliferation

Although this entity may occur both in the postoperative of the retinal scleral surgery and also independently of posterior segment surgery in cases of retinal detachment or proliferative diabetic retinopathy not surgically treated, this is described in this section, since diabetic patients with proliferative retinopathy are, perhaps, the most frequent with this complication, especially after posterior vitrectomy. Using ultrasound, the cyclitic membrane can be seen at the back of the iris plane with a shape of echogenic thickened band that encircles entirely the ocular globe in its most anterior portion. It is usually associated to the surrounding tractional retinal detachment extending from the ciliary body, giving a triangle shape of anterior base. A decreased production of aqueous humor is produced with prolonged hypotony that leads to a phthisis bulbi; we observe a choroidal thickening in ultrasound and a blood flow vanishing in Color-Doppler ultrasound (Fig. **6**).

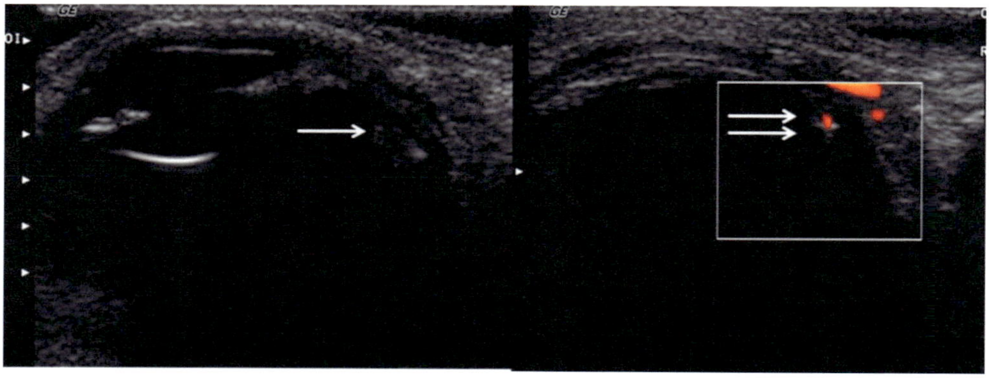

Figure 6: Sclerotomy new vessels [one arrow], vascularization is seen in color doppler [double arrow].

2. Ocular Hypotension

It is typical of 23 and 25 gauges sutureless surgeries; in sclerotomies, which are not closed with sutures, fluid can ooze to the subconjunctival space. The remaining of hypotension may cause a choroidal serous detachment, with the typical characteristics in ultrasound above mentioned.

3. Recurrent Vitreous Hemorrhage

Vitreous hemorrhage is one of the diseases that most often indicate the performance of posterior vitrectomy; its reappearance is caused by a surgical failure. The recurrence of hemorrhage is more common in processes like diabetic retinopathy, especially in its proliferative form, by being one of the most common causes of recurrence the appearance of new vesels at the sclerotomies level; these new vessels can be observed by Color-Doppler ultrasound, mainly, through a frequency of 20 MHz at the surgical sclerotomies level (Fig. **6**).

4. Retinal Detachment

In the posterior vitrectomy's postoperative and as a result of exerted tractions on the peripheral retina by the instruments, there may appear a retinal detachment; this presents the largest extension covering the entire retina many times as the main feature in vitrectomized patients; and it is also characteristic that the detachment occurs abruptly in a short space of time. Its ultrasonic features are not different from those of the rhegmatogenous detachment, previously described; although, we must remember that there is a vitreous absence in these cases, by showing a high mobility of the retina in the kinetic ultrasound.

OCULAR ULTRASOUND AND INNER TAMPONNADE

1. Liquid Perfluorocarbons

The use of liquid perfluorocarbons allows us to reapply the detached retina in the course of the vitrectomy, but it should be removed entirely at the end of it; if this does not happen, we are able to see the perfluorocarbon liquid remnants in the form of a highly echogenic area of lower level in the postoperative period. If the patient is in a sitting position, we see that these echoes occur at the bottom of the ocular globe while the rest of the globe remains with normal appearance; by lying down the patient, the highly echogenic area moves towards the ocular posterior pole, and this is due to the specific larger weight presented by the perfluorocarbon liquids. Therefore, the absence of perfluorocarbon liquid is essential if we want to study these patients by ultrasound. If there are liquid remnants, we can use an MRI to correctly visualize the ocular structures (Fig. **7**).

2. Perfluorocarbon Gases

The expanding gases are used in retinal detachment and macular holes surgeries after the practice of posterior vitrectomy; its function is of internal tamponnade while the scarring of tears or holes occurs being responsible for retinal detachment. Currently, the most widely used are SF6 and C3F8. By exploring the gas-filled eyes with ultrasound, we can see that the same gas prevents the ultrasound passage making impossible to observe any eye characteristic with the ultrasound. If the gas bubble fills the entire vitreous cavity, it is able to start looking at the ocular globe only when the gas begins to be reabsorbed. When the part of the gas is vanished, a mixed image is obtained by ultrasound in which the occupied part by the gas is highly echogenic preventing its exploration, and the free gas part has the usual looks in the ultrasound. We must, therefore, change the position of the head in order to explore the eye socket, and we must vary the patient position from right lateral decubitus to left lateral decubitus, sitting position, and submento-vertical position [Hirtz position] to allow the study of the different quadrants of the eye. Through these procedures, we can begin to examine patients from 24 to 48 hours after surgery.

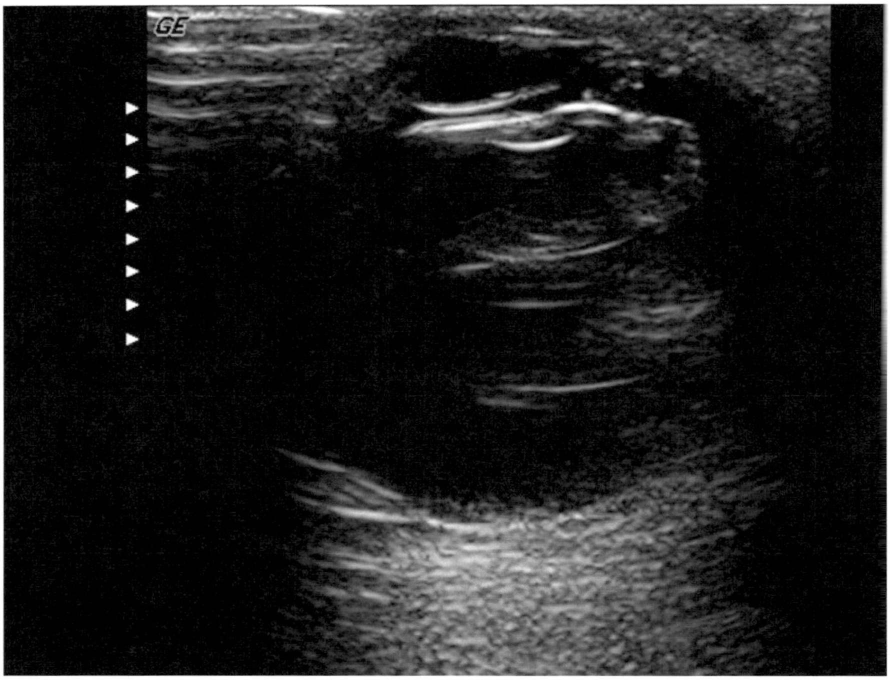

Figure 7: Ultrasound in a patient with intraocular silicon oil, the multiples echoes difficult the correct fundus vision.

3. Silicone Oil

The use of silicone oil is useful, at the end of the posterior segment surgery with vitrectomy, to maintain a long-term internal tamponnade in those patients with complicated retinal detachment, which by the use of gas we would not manage the retinal application. Silicone oils of 1000 or 5000 centistokes are used in these patients. The practice of echography in patients with silicone oil inside the ocular globe is totally impossible to perform, due to the high echogenicity of the oils preventing to see any ocular structure (Fig. 7); in these cases, we must resort to magnetic resonance imaging to visualize the ocular structures (Fig. 7). There may remain very small bubbles in the vitreous cavity in patients in whom the silicone oil have been removed from the eye socket; bubbles that we are able to see on ultrasound as small highly reflective echoes in the form of spicules, usually located in the ciliary processes area or the anterior chamber.

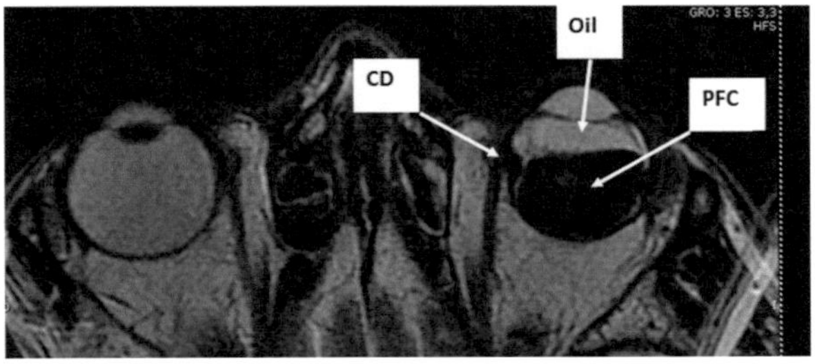

Figure 8: Complicated vitrectomy surgery, we can observe: Silicon oil (Oil), Liquid perfluorocarbon (PFC) and choroid detachment (CD).

ULTRASOUND IN POSTOPERATIVE ENDOPHTHALMITIS

Postoperative endophthalmitis is the eye infection occurring after an eye surgery that has required the opening of the eye [cataract, posterior vitrectomy, trabeculectomy, *etc.*], and the one that has allowed to pass the disease germs into it. The infection affects all the ocular structures observing the appearance of inflammatory cells and proteins at the aqueous humor and vitreous level, which may be seen as an important vitreitis preventing visualize the retina correctly. Endophthalmitis that appear between the second and the fifth day after surgery may be acute; subacute, appearing between the seventh and the 30th days postoperatively [some authors question its existence]; and chronic, taking place from the month of surgery.

ACUTE ENDOPHTHALMITIS

Using ultrasound, we can see the ultrasound translation of the aqueous Tyndall at the level of the anterior chamber in the form of not much echogenic thin dots diffusely distributed in the anterior chamber; by progressively appearing fibrin membranes, these appear as more echogenic threads (Fig. **9**). At the level of the vitreous cavity, we are able to observe a rise of the vitreous echogenicity that increases with the appearance of echogenic membranes giving a more heterogeneity aspect. If there is a posterior vitreous detachment, this can be delimited by observing a higher echogenicity of the posterior hyaloid. At the level of the eye wall, the choroid is clearly thickened (Fig. **9**). In these cases, it is important to rule out the presence of associated retinal detachment; in fact, the usefulness of echography in eyes with endophthalmitis is able to discard the detachment.

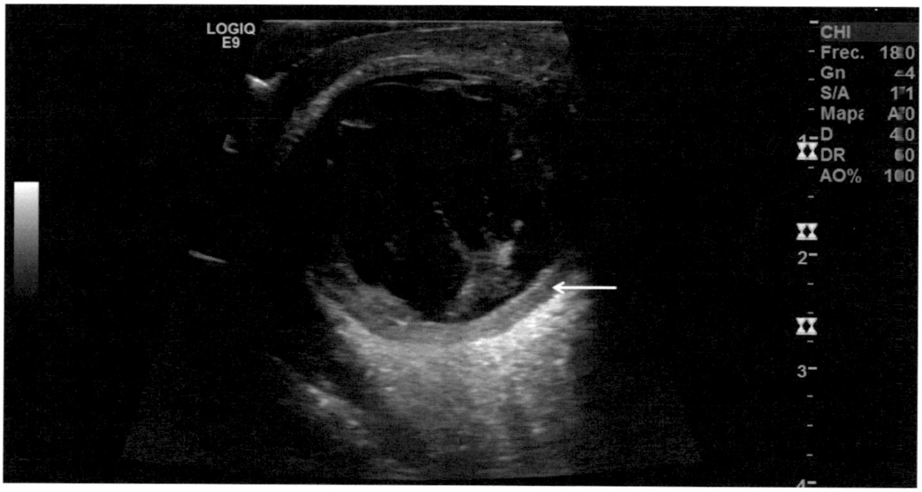

Figure 9: Vitreous body tracts in a case of endophthalmitis, with choroid thickening [white arrow].

CHRONIC ENDOPHTHALMITIS

In these cases, the obtained images do not differ from those in the chronic inflammatory process affecting the posterior segment [uveitis]. Thus, we can see the ultrasound translation of the aqueous Tyndall at the level of the anterior chamber in the form of not much echogenic thin dots diffusely distributed in the anterior chamber; in these patients, membrane formation more frequent at the anterior chamber level than in the acute form due to the chronification of the process. So, it is common to observe the fibrin membranes in the ultrasound; they appear as echogenic threads. At the vitreous cavity level, the observed heterogeneity in the ultrasound is higher than those of the acute processes, given the frequent occurrence of clearer vitreous membranes and gaps, giving multiple echoes in the vitreous cavity.

CONCLUDING REMARKS

The echography is an important technique in patients submitted to ocular surgery. In the preoperatory, the echography is mandatory if media opacities exist. In the postoperatory the difficulty to visualize ocular fundus is common; in these cases the echography helps to determine the presence of postoperative complications as retinal detachment, or suprachoroidal hemorrhage. In many of these instances the echography helps to indicate the moment of a second surgery; as in the case of suprachoroidal hemorrhage, the surgery becomes necessary when the hemorrhage clot becomes liquid, which usually happens in seven days, but it is only through echography that we determine the presence of liquid in the clot. The presence of perfluotrocarbon liquid in postoperative vitrectomy is useful in order to submit the patient to a second surgery. Despite the fact that echography has some limits and in the case of the presence of silicone oil, the ocular ultrasound has made a lot of artifacts which make the visualization of posterior segment difficult.

ACKNOWLEDGEMENTS

Declared None.

CONFLICT OF INTEREST

The authors confirm that this chapter contents have no conflict of interest.

REFERENCES

[1] Fong CS, Mitchell P, Rochtchina E, *et al.* Correction of visual impairment by cataract surgery and improved survival in older persons: the Blue Mountains Eye Study cohort. Ophthalmology. 2013; 120(9): 1720-7.

[2] Klein BE, Howard KP, Lee KE, *et al.* The relationship of cataract and cataract extraction to age-related macular degeneration: the Beaver Dam Eye Study. Ophthalmology. 2012; 119(8): 1628-33.

[3] Kahn HA, Leibowitz HM, Ganley JP, *et al.* The Framingham Eye Study. I. Outline and major prevalence findings. Am J Epidemiol. 1977; 106(1): 17-32.

[4] McCarty CA. Cataract in the 21st Century: lessons from previous epidemiological research. Clin Exp Optom. 2002; 85(2): 91-6.

[5] Tan AC, Loon SC, Choi H, *et al.* Lens Opacities Classification System III: cataract grading variability between junior and senior staff at a Singapore hospital. J Cataract Refract Surg. 2008; 34(11): 1948-52.

[6] Fielding JA. Imaging the eye with ultrasound.Br J Hosp Med. 1992 Jun 3-16; 47(11): 805-15.

[7] Bedi DG, Gombos DS, Ng CS, *et al.* Echography of the eye. AJR Am J Roentgenol. 2006; 187(4): 1061-72.

[8] Feretis E, Mourtzoukos S, Mangouritsas G, *et al.* Secondary management and outcome of massive suprachoroidal hemorrhage. Eur J Ophthalmol. 2006; 16(6): 835-40.

[9] Jin W, Xing Y, Xu Y, *et al.* Management of delayed suprachoriodal hemorrhage after intraocular surgery and trauma. Graefes Arch Clin Exp Ophthalmol. 2014 Jan 29.

[10] Lim LT, Agarwal PK, Rotchford A. Angle-closure glaucoma due to suprachoroidal hemorrhage secondary to disseminated intravascular coagulation. Semin Ophthalmol. 2011; 26(2): 59-60.

[11] Kaiser HJ, Shötzau A, Stümpfig D, *et al*. Blood flow velocities of the extraocular vessels in patients with high-tension and normal-tension primary open-angle glaucoma. Am J Ophthalmol 1997; 123: 320.

[12] Rankin SJ. Color-Doppler imaging of the retrobulbar circulation in glaucoma. Surv Ophthalmol. 1999; 43 Suppl 1: S176-82.

[13] Zvornicanin J, Jusufovic V, Cabric E, *et al*. Significance of echography in evaluation of vitreo-retinal pathologies. Med Arh. 2012; 66(5): 318-20.

CHAPTER 9

Ultrasound Compared to Other Ocular Imaging Systems

Pedro Romero-Aroca[1,*], Manuel Montero-Jaime[2,*], Marc Baget-Bernaldiz[1] and Victor Perez-Riverole[2]

[1]Department of Ophthalmology [2], Department of Radiology, University Hospital Sant Joan, Rovira & Virgili University, Pere Virgili Health Research Institute, IISPV, Reus, Spain

Abstract: Ophthalmology in the last decades has seen a great rise in new images techniques. The appearance of fluorescein angiography, optical tomography, *etc.* Highlight that other image techniques are unnecessary. But in fact in the present years, the ocular echography has become important, and the advances with new probes with higher frequencies, has helped us in a lot of ocular pathologies, as seen in the last chapter. In the present chapter we describe the indications of other image techniques used in medicine, but with poor knowledge in ophthalmology. The authors describe the indications of computer tomography and magnetic resonance, and also define when we use each technique.

Keywords: Computer tomography, magnetic resonance, choroid tumors, retinoblastoma, ocular calcifications, intraocular foreign body.

INTRODUCTION

In this chapter, we describe the ultrasound usefulness in the preoperative and postoperative diagnosis of various ocular entities prone to surgery, by dividing the different pathologies according to the ocular segment affected. Many of the entities described in this chapter have been previously described in other chapters; so in these, the descriptions are brief and refer to corresponding chapters. In this chapter, we emphasize the observed alterations by computed tomography and magnetic resonance imaging; diagnostic applications of computerized tomography and magnetic resonance imaging in the pathology of the ocular globe. Although the CT and the MRI are not seen as first-line imaging techniques in the diagnosis of intraocular pathology, there is no doubt that these represent complementary ultrasound techniques, especially in traumatic pathology and in tumors cases [1-4].

***Corresponding author Manuel Montero-Jaime:** Hospital Universitario Sant Joan, Avda. Doctor Josep Laporte 1 Reus, Spain; E-mail: mmontero@grupsagessa.com
Pedro Romero Aroca: Hospital Universitario Sant Joan, Avda. Doctor Josep Laporte 1 Reus, Spain; E-mail: pormero@grupsagessa.com

Pedro Romero-Aroca and Manuel Montero-Jaime (Eds.)

Overall, the lesions of thickness minor than 2 mm are not detected by CT or MRI. The MRI at High-Field, both 1.5 and 3 Tesla, is an imaging technique, thanks to the spatial resolution and tissue characterization that allow the identification of many diseases of the ocular globe and, essentially, the extraocular, which escapes this publication purpose. The CT should be performed on all trauma cases, especially if foreign body and/or bone injuries are suspected. In this chapter, we will discuss the usefulness of both techniques in the different diseases emphasizing those in which there is broad consensus, but without excluding other entities because the technical improvements change the diagnostic algorithms.

INTRAOCULAR TUMORS

The intraocular tumors classification is the subject of another chapter; but for clarification purposes, we can establish the most frequent diagnosis in function of its localization:

- Choroid:
  - Melanoma.
  - Metastasis.
  - Lymphoma.
  - Hemangioma.
- Retina:
  - Retinoblastoma.
- Iris:
  - Medulloepithelioma.

1. Melanoma

It is the most common uveal tumor, and it can be primary or be developed on a prior nevus. The differential diagnosis is laid out with: hemangioma, nevus, choroidal detachment, choroidal cysts, neurofibroma, schwannoma, leiomyoma, ciliary body adenoma and adenocarcinoma, medulloepithelioma, metastasis, retinal detachment and disciform macular degeneration. The morphological characteristics are determined by both techniques showing an appearance shaped as: oval, "mushroom", plate, ring, asymmetric or diffuse [5]. In CT, it appears as lesions of high density, high and well defined in the basal study. More important in the diagnosis is the PET/CT imaging technique [6, 7] (Fig. **1**). MRI is the technique of choice both for its detection and to assess the extraocular extension. Most of the melanomas show high signal in T1 because the paramagnetic properties of melanin, and low in T2 due to its high cellularity, with enhancement after contrast administration (Figs. **2**, **3**). Fat suppression sequences may exaggerate the melanoma extraocular extension, especially in the extraocular musculature's insertion, which usually shows high signal in this sequence [8, 9]. Necrosis and hemorrhage are common in melanomas appearing as high signal on T2. Another aspect to consider is the possibility of noticeable extraocular extension with a scarce intraocular representation.

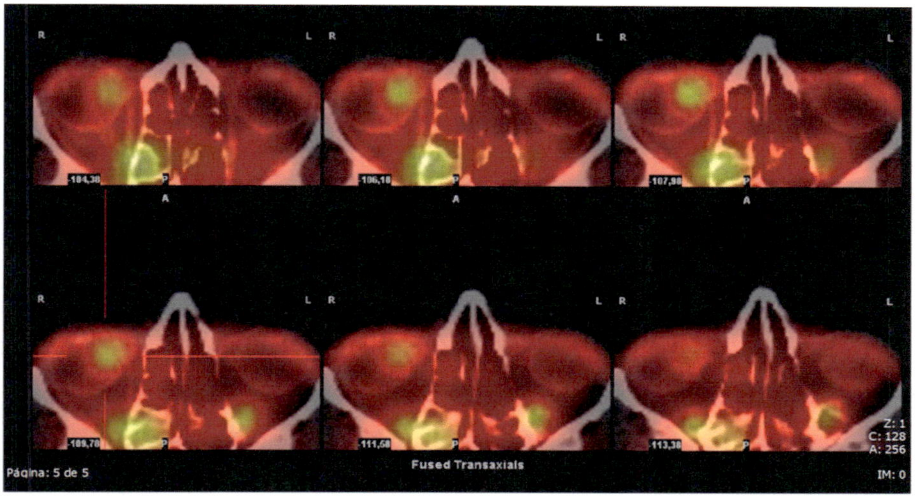

Figure 1: Choroidal melanoma in PET-CT.

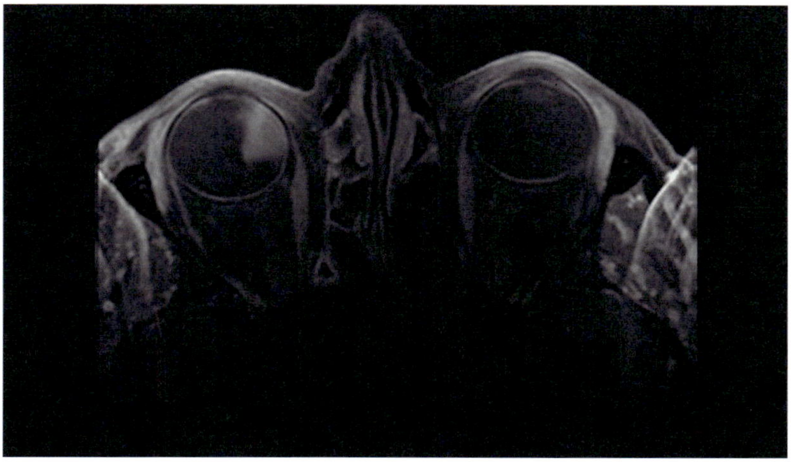

Figure 2: T1 magnetic resonance of choroidal melanoma.

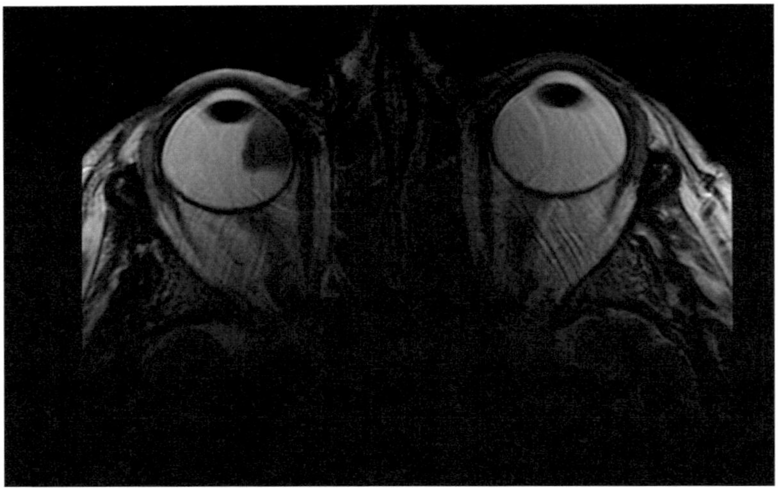

Figure 3: T2 magnetic resonance of choroidal melanoma.

2. Hemangiomas

They are congenital vascular hamartoma that may be solitary, usually in the posterior half of the eye; or multiple, in any location and in relation to the Sturge-Weber syndrome. Lesions appear on CT as high density with significant enhancement after contrast administration. The MRI shows well-defined isointense or slightly hyperintense lesions in relation to the vitreous in T1-sequences and markedly hyperintense on T2, by appearing isointense in relation to the vitreous. After administering a contrast agent, a noticeable relief is observed [10].

3. Choroidal Nevus

They are congenital lesions that can be detected at later times, like hemangiomas. As those, they are usually located in the posterior half of the ocular globe. Generally, they are less than 2 mm thick due to being flat lesions that are not detected on CT or MRI. When they exceed the 3 mm, the signal characteristics are identical to those of a melanoma.

4. Metastasis

Most of them are located in the posterior half of the ocular globe, since they reach the uvea by the posterior ciliary arteries. The MR signal behavior can be similar to melanoma, although its morphology is more flattened. Sometimes they are so small that they are barely detected, especially if there is associated RD.

5. Lymphoma and Leukaemia

The condition may be unilateral or bilateral. Usually, they show low signal on T1 and T2, especially in the case of lymphoma by its hypercellularity. After administering contrast agent, the relief is observed.

6. Retinoblastoma

Although many of these tumors show calcification [90%], and the CT is more sensitive than US and MRI for detection; the MRI is the technique of choice for the assessment of extraocular extension. In any child under 3 years, the presence of intraocular calcification should warn about the existence of a retinoblastoma. Another special feature of this tumor is the bilateralism and intracranial concomitant involvement, especially in the pineal region. They are lesions moderately hyperdense in the CT, with calcification and relief after the contrast agent. They show intermediate signal on T1 and low T2 signal in the MRI, with moderate relief after administering contrast agent [11].

7. Medulloepithelioma

These types of tumors are extremely rare in adults. In MRI, they behave as high signal lesions on T1 and low signal on T2, similar to the behavior of melanoma.

ANOTHER PSEUDOTUMORAL LESION

1. Age-Related Macular Degeneration

In many cases, it takes a pseudotumoral morphology. In CT, the appearance is similar to melanoma, but with greater relief after administering contrast agent. In MR, the appearance depends on the stage of the disease and, mainly, on the presence of hemorrhage, by varying from lesions of high signal on T1 and T2 in acute phase (Figs. **4**, **5**), with low signal on T1 and high T2 to in subacute lesions, and finally hypotensive in both T1 and T2, in chronic lesions; these last are indistinguishable from melanoma. After administering contrast agent, the relief is shown from moderate to noticeable.

2. Posterior Scleritis

The scleritis may be associated with infectious processes [bacterial, fungal or viral], metabolic processes as gout, and processes of autoimmune nature as rheumatoid arthritis, polyarteritis nodosa, SLE, and relapsing polychondritis. The posterior scleritis may be acute or chronic, and the result is a choroidal and scleral thickening [12] (Fig. **6**). There is a nodular form, granulomatous inflammatory variant, which is indistinguishable imaging of melanoma. The diffuse form shows ocular layers thickening with more or less homogeneous relief after administering contrast agent.

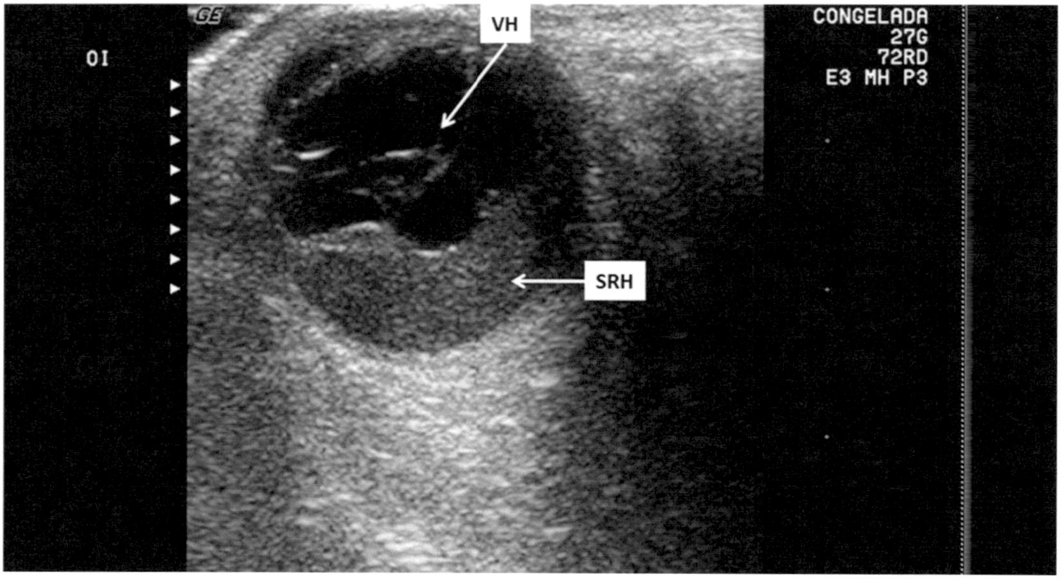

Figure 4: Subretinal hemorrhage (SRH) in a patient with age related macular degeneration, with vitreous hemorrhage (VH).

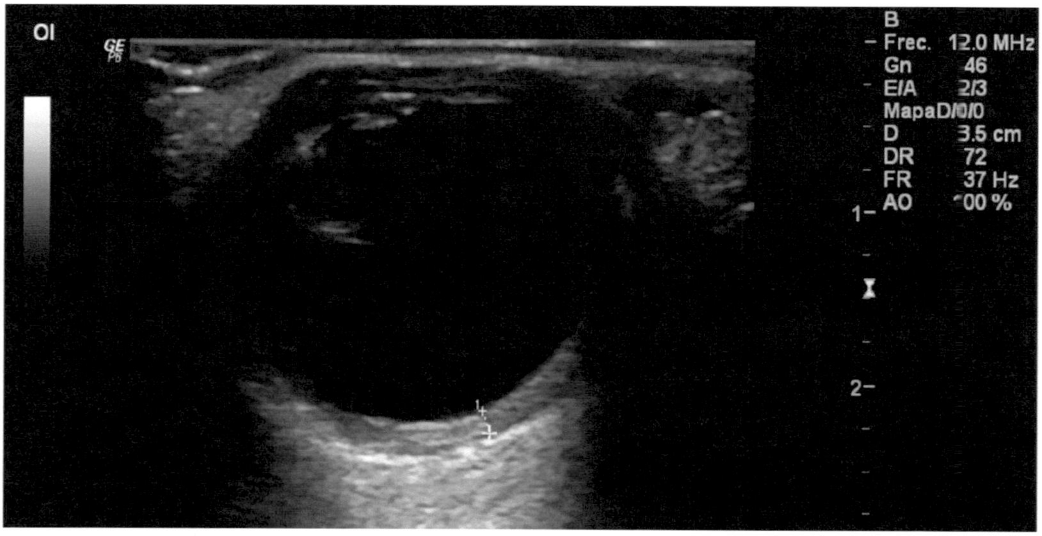

Figure 5: Posterior scleritis, thickened posterior sclera, market with asterisks.

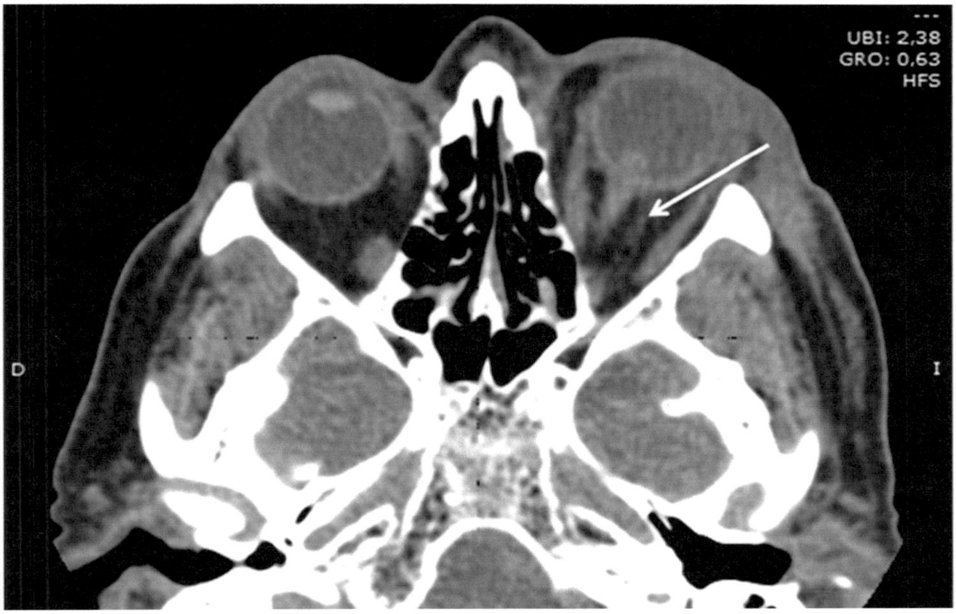

Figure 6: Fat rarefication (White arrow) between optic nerve and lateral rectus muscle in TC.

CALCIFICATIONS

The technique of choice for its evaluation is the TC. The intraocular calcifications occur in physiologically way, usually associated with age and muscle attachments, or in connection with infectious, inflammation, trauma and tumor pathologies, mainly the retinoblastoma and the teratoid variety medulloepithelioma. Also, the chronic retinal detachments are able to calcify. The choroidal osteoma is an infrequent and well-defined benign tumor, and it is detected incidentally in young women. It has a unilateral or bilateral parapapillary location. In the cytomegalovirus retinitis associated with HIV infection, the calcifications are frequent. Another common cause of intraocular calcification is the drusen. Due to their size, the drusen located in the retina avoids the imaging techniques, both US and MRI or CT [13]. In contrast, those located in relation to the optic nerve are easily valuables with CT. Finally, we have to consider the trauma as a common cause of calcification, usually delayed in time.

ENDOPHTHALMITIS

It is a non-infectious inflammatory or infectious process affecting the vitreous chamber and/or anterior chamber after surgery, trauma or systemic infection. The CT scan shows vitreous hyperdensity. In MRI, the increase of signal on T1 and

FLAIR is appreciated due to the presence of protein by the exudate [14-16]. After administering the contrast agent, we see uptake and uveal thickening with potential microabscesses. Retinal, choroidal and posterior vitreous detachment may be explored by both techniques, mainly MRI.

EYE TRAUMA

Developed in the corresponding chapter, we insist only on the need for CT in cases of ocular trauma, mainly in perforation cases or foreign body suspicion; in case of ocular globe posterior rupture, we see an orbitary fat reaction in the form of a fat rarefication. This finding is observed in Fig. **6** next to the globe between optic nerve and lateral muscle, the posterior rupture is suspected in ecography as a hypersignal in vitreous adjacent to rupture (Fig. **7**); despite only in this case the surgery by vitrectomy demonstrated the posterior globus rupture. In addition, if there is suspicion of bony orbital walls damage, the TC is preferred [17].

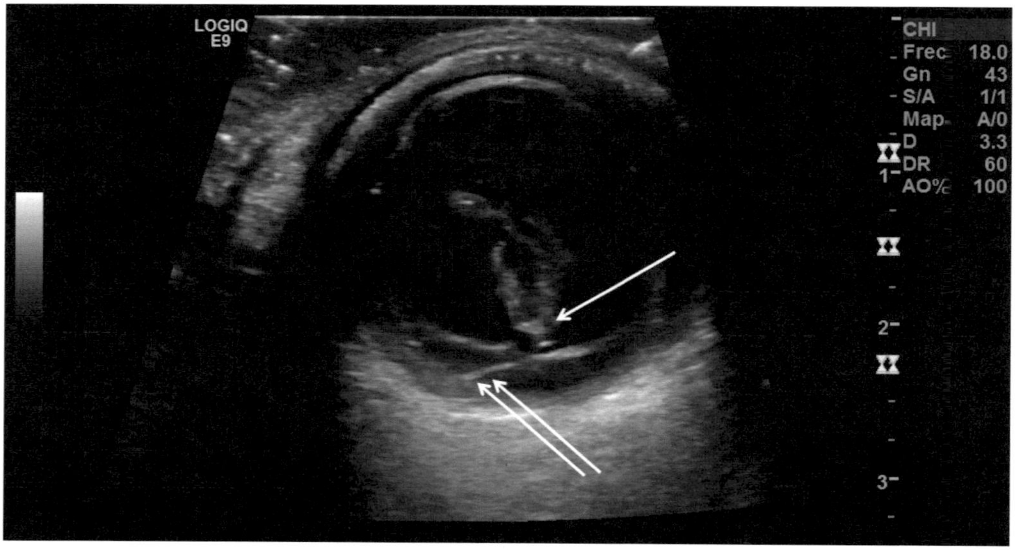

Figure 7: Vitreous rarefication [one arrow] in echography. The area of possible scleral rupture is signaled by double arrow.

CHOROIDAL DETACHMENT

It may be serous or hemorrhagic, and its causes have been described in the corresponding chapter. The image features, mainly in MRI, vary depending on the subchoroidal fluid composition [18, 19]. Thus, the hemorrhage is isointense or hypointense with the vitreous on T1; and markedly hypointense on T2, whether it is acute [0-48 hours]; hyperintense on T1 and hypointense on T2, whether it is early subacute; and of high signal on T1 and T2, whether it is subacute late-chronic [more than 3 weeks]. On the other hand, the exudates have a high signal on T1 due to the protein content. If they are morphologically complete, they show a biconvex morphology with an anterior extension beyond the ora serrata. The partial ones present a "hump" shape with well-defined contours.

RETINAL DETACHMENT

The signal characteristics are similar to those of the choroid depending on the subretinal fluid characteristics. If they are morphologically complete, they adopt morphology of funnel with the vertex at the optic disc and the anterior arms in the ora serrata. The coronal image shows the characteristic retinal folds. The most interesting aspect of MRI is the usefulness for the detection of pathology associated neoplastic and the assessing of the retina condition in patients treated with oily substances injection that hinder the ultrasonographic monitoring.

CONCLUDING REMARKS

Computer tomography and magnetic resonance are two techniques of great importance in ophthalmic examination. The intraocular tumors are the most important pathologies in which ultrasound examination are applied, but the magnetic resonance helps us in the diagnosis. Furthermore, the presence of calcification seen in computer tomography indicates a possible origin of the tumor. In ocular trauma the basic examination is done under CT if we suspect the presence of intraocular foreign body.

ACKNOWLEDGEMENTS

Declared None.

CONFLICT OF INTEREST

The authors confirm that this chapter contents have no conflict of interest.

REFERENCES

[1] Artmann H, Grau H, Losche CC. The significance of computed tomography in ophthalmologic diagnosis. I: The place of computed tomography, indications, study technics, anatomic representation, computed tomography of eyeball and orbital injuriesRadiol Diagn(Berl). 1989; 30(6): 621-8.

[2] Harlan JB Jr, Pieramici DJ. Evaluation of patients with ocular trauma. Ophthalmol Clin North Am. 2002; 15(2): 153-61.

[3] Joseph DP, Pieramici DJ, Beauchamp NJ Jr. Computed tomography in the diagnosis and prognosis of open-globe injuries. Ophthalmology. 2000; 107(10): 1899-906.

[4] Turbin RE, Maxwell DN, Langer PD, *et al.* Patterns of transorbital intracranial injury: a review and comparison of occult and non-occult cases.Surv Ophthalmol. 2006; 51(5): 449-60.

[5] Scott IU, Murray TG, Hughes JR. Evaluation of imaging techniques for detection of extraocular extension of choroidal melanoma. Arch Ophthalmol. 1998; 116(7): 897-9.

[6] Reddy S, Kurli M, Tena LB, *et al.* PET/CT imaging: detection of choroidal melanoma. Br J Ophthalmol. 2005; 89(10): 1265-9.

[7] Romero-Aroca P, Montero-Jaime M, Intriago B, *et al.* 18FDG-PET/CT assessing the absence of cell viability and excluding metastatic disease in a case of necrotic choroidal melanoma. Eur J Ophthalmol. 2012; 22(2): 288-92.

[8] Lemke AJ, Hosten N, Bornfeld N, *et al.* Appearance of choroidal melanoma on high resolution MRI using 1.5T with a dedicated surface coil in 200 consecutive patients). Rofo. 1998; 169(5): 47 -8.

[9] Lucignani G, Paganelli G, Modorati G, *et al.* MRI, antibody-guided scintigraphy, and glucose metabolism in uveal melanoma. J Comput Assist Tomogr. 1992; 16(1): 77-83.

[10] Stroszczynski C, Hosten N, Bornfeld N, *et al.* Choroidal hemangioma: MR findings and differentiation from uveal melanoma. Am J Neuroradiol. 1998; 19(8): 1441-7.

[11] Khurana A, Eisenhut CA, Wan W, *et al.* Comparison of the diagnostic value of MR imaging and ophthalmoscopy for the staging of retinoblastoma. Eur Radiol. 2013; 23(5): 1271-80.

[12] Mansour AM, Han DP, Kim JE, *et al.* Radiologic findings in infected and noninfected scleral buckles. Eur J Ophthalmol. 2007; 17(5): 804-11.

[13] Romani A, Baldeschi L, Genovesi-Ebert F, *et al.* Sensitivity and specificity of echography, fluorescein videoangiography, indocyanine green videoangiography, magnetic resonance and radioimmunoscintigraphy in the diagnosis of primary choroidal malignant melanoma. Ophthalmologica. 1998; 212 Suppl 1: 44-6.

[14] Rumboldt Z, Moses C, Wieczerzynski U, *et al.* Diffusion-weighted imaging, apparent diffusion coefficients, and fluid-attenuated inversion recovery MR imaging in endophthalmitis. AJNR Am J Neuroradiol. 2005; 26(7): 1869-72.

[15] Lee CC, Chen CY, Chen FH, *et al.* Septic metastatic endophthalmitis from Klebsiella pneumoniae liver abscess: CT and MR imaging characteristics--report of three cases. Radiology. 1998; 207(2): 411-6.

[16] Yu E, Laughlin S, Kassel EE, *et al.* Nocardial endophthalmitis and subretinal abscess: CT and MR imaging features with pathologic correlation: a case report. AJNR Am J Neuroradiol. 2005; 26(5): 1220-2.

[17] Kubal WS. The pathological globe: clinical and imaging analysis. Semin Ultrasound CT MR. 1997; 18(6): 423-36.

[18] Shellock FG, Crues JV. MR procedures: biologic effects, safety, and patient care. Radiology. 2004; 232(3): 635-52.

[19] Lustrin ES, Brown JH, Novelline R, *et al.* Radiologic assessment of trauma and foreign bodies of the eye and orbit.Neuroimaging Clin N Am. 1996; 6(1): 219-37.

Subject Index

Made in the USA
Las Vegas, NV
04 November 2026

57431560R00086